The Schwarzbein Principle
Vegetarian Cookbook

THE SCHWARZBEIN PRINCIPLE

Vegetarian

COOKBOOK

Diana Schwarzbein, M.D.
Nancy Deville
and Evelyn Jacob

Health Communications, Inc.
Deerfield Beach, Florida

www.hci-online.com

The Schwarzbein Principle Vegetarian Cookbook and the recipes within are not intended as a substitute for the advice and/or medical care of the reader's physician, nor are they meant to discourage or dissuade the reader from the advice of his or her physician. The reader should regularly consult with a physician in matters relating to his or her health, and especially with regard to symptoms that may require diagnosis. Any eating or lifestyle regimen should be undertaken under the direct supervision of the reader's physician. Moreover, anyone with chronic or serious ailments should undertake any eating and lifestyle program, and/or changes to his or her personal eating and lifestyle regimen under the direct supervision of his or her physician. If the reader has any questions concerning the information presented in this book, or its application to his or her particular medical profile, or if the reader has unusual medical or nutritional needs or constraints that may conflict with the advice in this book he or she should consult his or her physician. If the reader is pregnant or nursing she should consult her physician before embarking on any nutrition or lifestyle program.

Library of Congress Cataloging-in-Publication Data

Schwarzbein, Diana
    The Schwarzbein principle vegetarian cookbook / Diana Schwarzbein, Nancy Deville, and Evelyn Jacob.
      p.   cm.
    ISBN 1-55874-682-X
    1. Vegetarian cookery.   I. Deville, Nancy.   II. Jacob, Evelyn.   III. Title.
TX837.S324   1999   99-15011
641.5'636—dc21   CIP

ISBN 1-55874-682-X

Publisher: Health Communications, Inc.
              3201 S.W. 15th Street
              Deerfield Beach, FL 33442-8190

R-05-02

Cover design by Lisa Camp

For my papi,
Z. Edison Schwarzbein, Ph.D.,
for his love and guidance.

—Diana Schwarzbein, M.D.

For my grandma,
Estelle Grabowski, who always said
an egg was the perfect food.

—Nancy Deville

For Arno, Joss, Bowie and Malia
with my deepest love
and gratitude.

—Evelyn Jacob

Contents

Acknowledgments

This cookbook is the direct result of a deluge of requests by readers of *The Schwarzbein Principle*. Many, many thanks to our enthusiastic supporters.

We are indebted to a number of people who worked on this project. We are grateful to those who contributed recipes and ideas. We thank Adele Staal, Sheridan Eldridge and all the volunteers from Project Food Chain for experimenting with recipes and giving feedback.

Orien Armstrong, was, as always, a pleasure to work with. David Stanley and Harold "Wardie" Ward gave much-needed computer support. A special thanks to Kelli Tatlock who has been an invaluable assistant during the writing of this book—and for always being cheerful.

From Diana Schwarzbein, M.D., thank you to all my patients for sticking to the program without the benefit of recipes.

From Nancy, sincere thanks to Pat Frederick for her superb editorial skills, attention, support and endurance in the face of unending details—and for being a pleasure to work with. Thanks to Joy Morrison, Reneé Perez and Jillian Jacobs at The Owner Managed Business Institute for clerical support.

From Evelyn, thanks to Joss and Bowie for being such fans of Momma's cooking, and to my culinary inspirations and special friends, Julia Child and Don "Skip" Skipworth, who have enriched my life.

The *Schwarzbein Principle Cookbooks* would not have been published if not for Russell Bishop who introduced us to Jack Canfield who, in turn, gave our manuscripts to Peter Vegso at Health Communications, Inc. We are grateful to Peter for believing in our project, and for his infectious enthusiasm. Many thanks to our agent, Barbara Neighbors Deal, for handling the details that went into making our publishing deal.

Peter's staff at HCI made the final editorial process so painless, we actually enjoyed it. We give special acknowledgment to: Christine Belleris, editorial codirector, and Allison Janse, associate editor, who were there with us through thick and thin; Kim Weiss and Maria Konicki in PR; Lisa Camp for the cover design; Erica Orloff for an excellent job copyediting; Lawna Oldfield for the inside book design; Susan Olason for the index; and Teri Peluso, executive assistant, for all of their expertise, support and hard work in getting the book to press.

We also thank Lisa Ekus and Merrilyn Lewis at Lisa Ekus Public Relations for their wonderful efforts on our behalf.

But most of all we are grateful to our husbands, Larry Mousouris, John Davis and Arno Jaffe for their love, patience, understanding and *appetites*.

Introduction

Americans are in constant pursuit of good health. We are deluged with information on how to improve eating and lifestyle habits. We look to "healthier" cultures for the answers. The French, rural Chinese, Inuits, Africans and Tibetans have all been examined in an attempt to understand why they do not suffer the same high rate of chronic degenerative diseases as we do in this country.

The so-called "French paradox" implies that the lower rate of heart disease in the French population, despite their high-fat intake, can be attributed to the fact that they drink wine. That must mean drinking a lot of wine is good for you. But the Inuits eat a *high*-fat diet. It must be the fish oils. We need to eat more fish. Africans eat wild game, which is high in saturated fats. But of course they exercise more than we do. We must exercise more. What about the Tibetans, who drink yak-butter tea all day long? Could it be the altitude?

All of these conclusions seem plausible—especially if you still believe that eating a low-fat diet is healthy. But consider the common denominator in these four cultures: The French, Inuits, Africans and Tibetans all eat a diet of "real" foods—foods that they could, in theory, pick, gather or milk. But equally important: *They eat foods that are rich in good fats.* In other words, these cultures have remained the healthiest in the world because they have *not* gone on low-fat diets.

If you have read *The Schwarzbein Principle* you know why eating a low-fat diet, high in carbohydrates and stimulants, is the major factor in the rise in chronic degenerative diseases in our country.

What You Will Learn When You Read *The Schwarzbein Principle*

Prolonged high insulin levels set off a multitude of chain reactions that disrupt all other hormones and biochemical reactions at the cellular level. This chronic disruption, termed "accelerated metabolic aging," leads to body-fat gain, chronic conditions and degenerative diseases. The factors that raise insulin levels, both directly and indirectly are: eating a low-fat, high-carbohydrate diet, stress, dieting, caffeine, alcohol, aspartame (an artificial sweetener), tobacco, steroids, stimulant and other recreational drugs, lack of exercise, excessive and/or unnecessary thyroid replacement therapy and all over-the-counter and prescription drugs. These factors have become central in the eating and lifestyle habits that have prevailed over the last twenty years and that parallel the rise in the incidence of disease during this same period of time.

The Schwarzbein program, which includes balanced nutrition, stress management, exercise, the elimination of stimulants and other drugs, and hormone replacement therapy, if needed, is a complete program designed to balance insulin and all other hormone levels. Anyone can prevent accelerated aging and disease, achieve ideal body composition and extend longevity by following this program.

In addition to drastically limiting fats from our diets, since the Industrial Revolution most people have stopped eating foods found in nature. People now eat invented, chemically altered or created substances we call "products." We tend to think that our bodies will simply process anything we put in them. But every single thing that goes into our mouths should be used as building material or energy. If it is not it is perceived by our bodies as a dangerous substance. Products like saccharine, margarine and other invented substances, along with refined and processed foods, are harmful substances to human physiology. Because chemical processes proceed on a molecular level, we must think about what we put into our bodies. In fact, since we have stopped eating foods found in nature, we must think about what we ingest even more.

To keep up the replenishing process within the human body, proteins and fats are the most important of the essential nutrient groups. In addition to making structures (bones, nails, hair), proteins and fats are necessary for the formation of all the chemicals needed for survival, such as hormones, enzymes and neurotransmitters. Nonstarchy vegetables are useful as a source of vitamins, minerals and fiber. Carbohydrates are used mainly to fuel the body, like gasoline for a car. Besides providing these materials and energy, *the four nutrient groups need to be eaten together to balance all the hormone systems of the body.*

Balanced Nutrition

The healing-and-maintenance eating programs (explained in detail in *The Schwarzbein Principle*) are not just one more fad diet that advocates eliminating one or two of the nutrient groups. You should *not* stop eating carbohydrates, or even drastically reduce carbohydrates in your diet. *This is not a high-fat, high-protein, low-carbohydrate diet.* It is a balanced nutritional program tailored to improve each individual's specific metabolism. Not eating enough carbohydrates is just as harmful as eating too many. The key to this program is determining your individual carbohydrate need. To do this *you must eat from the four basic nutrient groups* and you must eat the quantity of real carbohydrates (not man-made) that match your activity level, current health and metabolism.

Many people who eat a vegetarian diet believe that if they do not eat meat, fish or poultry, they are eating well. The typical vegetarian breakfast consists of shredded wheat, soy milk, fruit, orange juice, black coffee; salad with an unbuttered roll for lunch; and pasta with marinara sauce and a glass of wine for dinner. This diet is designed to avoid animal products and fats and is high in carbohydrates, which to many may seem ideal. But if you have read *The Schwarzbein Principle* you know that nothing can be more damaging to your health than a high-carbohydrate, low-protein, low-fat diet! What is even worse is that, along with a high-carbohydrate, low-protein, low-fat diet, people are eating processed foods (cereal, bread, pasta) and ingesting stimulants (coffee, wine).

People who follow a vegetarian diet do not set out to become unhealthy. On the contrary, the majority of vegetarians are health conscious—but they have been given the wrong information. The good news is that eating a vegetarian diet *is* healthy if followed properly.

However, many people either do not know how to cook, do not like to cook or do not have time to cook. With that in mind, we decided to go beyond the meal plans included in *The Schwarzbein Principle* and provide readers with easily accessible recipes to launch a new healthy lifestyle. We looked for an experienced cook who could compile our cookbooks. Evelyn Jacob, who had culinary expertise in preparing "Schwarzbein" meals, was a natural choice. The delicious recipes she created for this cookbook are both "gourmet" and easy enough for inexperienced cooks to prepare. For those who eat a vegetarian diet, it is essential to put back the proteins and fats that have been inadvertently eliminated from their diet. Since it is impossible to get enough protein from non-animal sources without eating too many carbohydrates, Evelyn's recipes are "ovo-lacto," including cheese and eggs.

We owe a debt of gratitude to "The Schwarzbein Principle Chef," Evelyn Jacob, who not only has an innate sense about food and a talent for cooking but who also met the challenge of this project with a can-do attitude and a high degree of professionalism.

This cookbook is the perfect guide for all of you who want to follow The Schwarzbein Program.

Bon Appetit!

Diana Schwarzbein, M.D.
Nancy Deville

Before You Begin Cooking

Eat Enough Food

Be sure to eat as much protein, fat and nonstarchy vegetables as you want. However, everyone needs a different amount of carbohydrates depending on current health, metabolism and activity level. The recipes in this book are both for those on the Healing Program and the Maintenance Program as described in *The Schwarzbein Principle*. Carbohydrate grams vary from recipe to recipe.

It is very important to eat enough food. When you reduce your carbohydrate consumption, you *must* increase proteins, fats and nonstarchy vegetables. Eating enough food is the only way to heal your metabolism and get off the accelerated metabolic aging track.[1]

Combine Recipes to Create Balanced Meals

The vegetarian diet is more limited than a meat-based diet. Many who eat a vegetarian diet do not want to eat soy products or eggs at every meal. But, if you limit protein at the same time that you limit carbohydrates, you will not eat enough food in some of your meals. It is

---

[1]*Accelerated metabolic aging is explained in detail in* The Schwarzbein Principle.

important to balance your meals with proteins, fats, nonstarchy vegetables and carbohydrates. Some of the recipes in this book contain a higher amount of carbohydrates than some people should eat at one meal. To eat a balanced diet of all the essential nutrient groups, you must combine recipes. For example, if a recipe contains too many carbohydrates for you, then reduce the serving size and eat it along with a main-course protein dish.

Nutritional Analysis

To help you prepare balanced meals, each recipe in this book has been analyzed and is accompanied by an approximate breakdown of protein and carbohydrate grams. These totals do not necessarily account for every carbohydrate present in each ingredient. The reason is that some recipes contain foods, such as nonstarchy vegetables, that have a low glycemic index so you can eat as much of them as you want.[2] Heavy cream, butter and other good fats also alter the glycemic index and therefore lower the number of carbohydrates in some recipes. You may notice that some recipes containing nonstarchy vegetables still show some carbohydrate. The reason is these recipes contain an ingredient, such as tomato paste, that has a higher glycemic index.

Occasionally a recipe will list a food, such as brown rice, that will not be included in the serving portion analysis. In this case, the analysis of that food will be noted separately. If not noted, then all ingredients were analyzed to come up with protein and carbohydrate grams per serving.

Fat grams are not included in the analysis, both because you should not count fat grams, and more important, you should eat as much good fat as your body needs.

---

[2] *The glycemic index is explained in detail in* The Schwarzbein Principle.

Why You Do Not Need to Salt Your Foods

Our recipes do not call for salt because natural foods contain enough sodium. Eating excess salt unnecessarily strains your kidneys, contributing to the accelerated metabolic aging process. If you desire optimal health, you must slowly wean yourself from using salt. As you decrease your salt intake you may go through an adjustment period while you become used to the taste of food without added salt. Eventually you will be able to fully appreciate the *real* taste of food. And, more important, you will be one step closer to your goal of optimal health and an ideal body composition.

A Few Other Helpful Tips

• It is essential that you read *The Schwarzbein Principle* to fully understand the importance of a balanced diet comprised of all the essential nutrient groups: proteins, fats, nonstarchy vegetables and carbohydrates.

• Before cooking, read the following section, "All You Need to Know About Tofu."

• Some of our recipes call for low-sodium tamari soy sauce, which does contain some salt and therefore should be used sparingly.

• Be sure to check cream containers so that you buy "all-dairy" cream. Avoid using cream or any other product containing chemical additives.

• Use real, unsalted butter. Never eat margarine or any other hydrogenated fat.

• Always buy the freshest foods possible. Use foods in their whole state—real foods that you could, in theory, pick, gather or milk from an animal. Whenever possible, buy organically grown produce and grains.

- Always use whole plain yogurt and whole sour cream. Do not use low-fat or any other processed food products.

- Use only pure-pressed oils. Use mayonnaise made from pure-pressed canola oil.

- A few recipes call for small amounts of flour, which is a processed food and should not be eaten regularly. Whenever possible, use whole-grain flour.

- Occasionally you will see a recipe that calls for small amounts of orange juice. Juices are high in carbohydrates and should always be consumed as part of a balanced meal.

- Some recipes call for small amounts of alcohol. While alcohol is a stimulant and should be avoided, you can use small amounts in recipes because most of the alcohol evaporates during cooking.

- If you purchase sauces or any other products, make sure to check for sugar-free, chemical-free products.

- Thoroughly wash all vegetables and fruits before using.

- To clean mushrooms, wipe them with a damp cloth.

- To sliver fresh basil, remove leaves from stems, rinse in cold water, roll leaves into a cigar-like tube and cut into fine slivers. (This process avoids bruising the delicate leaves.)

- To finely mince fresh ginger, peel ginger with a sharp knife or peeler, cut into thin slices and finely mince.

- If you are concerned about salmonella, do not use the recipes that call for raw eggs.

All You Need to Know About Tofu

If you eat a vegetarian diet you must focus on getting adequate protein in each and every meal. For that reason, tofu, a complete vegetable protein, is often the staple of a balanced vegetarian diet.

Tofu, an excellent source of calcium and iron, is high in protein, low in carbohydrates and is easy to digest.

Tofu is economical and can be found in most supermarkets. There are three common varieties of tofu: soft, medium and firm. Our recipes use firm tofu, since it has the highest amount of protein and the most flavor. Tofu has the reputation for being "bland," but if you follow the directions for preparing tofu you will find that it absorbs marinades well, and, when prepared with other flavorful foods, it complements and enhances many recipes.

You can find tofu packaged so that it does not need refrigeration, or in sealed containers in the refrigerated section of your market. Either way, be sure to check the expiration date. Once you have opened either type of packaging, it is best to rinse the tofu and transfer it to a jar with a tight-fitting lid. Change the water every other day. Tofu should have a sweet smell. When it is spoiled, it feels slimy and has a sour odor. Even though tofu may keep for over a week or two, it is always best to eat all foods as fresh as possible.

Two important techniques rid tofu of its blandness and maximize its subtle flavor. First, take the tofu out of its packaging and pour off the water. Rinse in fresh water, then slice lengthwise into halves or thirds. Place the drained tofu in a shallow, flat pan. Slant the pan by propping up one edge to allow moisture to drain away. Drape a clean dishtowel over the tofu and set a heavy casserole filled with water on top to act as a weight, pressing out the excess moisture. Let the tofu drain thirty minutes.

Next, marinate the tofu for several hours or days until it "gives up" its blandness and takes on the flavor of the marinade. Prepare a marinade of your choice or use the following basic recipe. When tofu is drained and marinated, it can be grilled, baked or sautéed. Enjoy the wonderful flavor of this unique food.

Basic Marinated Tofu

Makes 6 servings • Each serving: 26 grams protein • 7 grams carbohydrate

2 pounds firm tofu, drained, pressed and sliced crosswise into 4 slabs (for directions, see "All You Need to Know About Tofu," page 10)

½ ounce dried shitake or porcini mushrooms

1 cup hot water

2 minced garlic cloves

2 teaspoons peeled and finely minced fresh ginger

½ cup rice wine vinegar

½ cup pure-pressed sesame oil

¼ cup low-sodium tamari soy sauce

2 tablespoons fresh lime juice

dash cayenne pepper

2 tablespoons minced scallions

2 tablespoons minced fresh cilantro

Prepare tofu and set aside. Immerse mushrooms in hot water and soak 15 minutes. Remove from water. Slice off and discard hard stem nubs and slice mushrooms into thin slivers. Strain the liquid that mushrooms have been soaking in through a fine sieve lined with a paper towel, and save for a future soup stock.

In a medium bowl, combine slivered mushrooms, garlic, ginger, rice wine vinegar, sesame oil, soy sauce, lime juice, cayenne pepper, scallions and cilantro. Mix well with a fork. Pour over tofu. Store covered in the refrigerator. Marinate 1 hour to 2 days, turning occasionally.

Preheat oven to 375°. Remove tofu from marinade, arrange on a greased baking sheet and bake about 30 minutes, turning once. Pour marinade into a small saucepan and simmer until hot. Serve on the side with the baked tofu.

Quick and Easy Methods of Preparing Tofu

Broiling: Preheat broiler. Arrange drained and marinated tofu on a greased rack with a tinfoil-lined baking sheet underneath. Broil about 5 minutes on each side. Serve immediately.

Baking: Preheat oven to 375°. Arrange drained and marinated tofu on a greased baking sheet. Bake about 30 minutes, turning occasionally, until evenly browned. Serve immediately.

Sautéing: In a large nonstick skillet, heat 2 tablespoons pure-pressed extra virgin olive oil over medium-high heat. When oil is hot, add drained and marinated tofu and sauté about 5 minutes on each side, or until evenly browned, stirring occasionally. Serve immediately.

Breakfast Entrées

Assorted Entrées

Frittatas and Fabulous Variations

Omelets

Scrambled Eggs

Scrambled Tofu

Smoothies

Assorted Entrées

Annette Matrisciano's Cheesy Eggs

Makes 2 servings • Each serving: 25 grams protein • 2 grams carbohydrate

4 eggs

3 ounces cream cheese, cut into
 ½-inch cubes

¼ cup grated Parmesan cheese

freshly ground black pepper,
 to taste

1½ tablespoons unsalted butter

1 minced garlic clove

In a small bowl, beat eggs with cream-cheese cubes, Parmesan cheese and black pepper. Set aside.

In a medium nonstick skillet, melt butter over medium-high heat. When butter is hot and bubbly, add garlic and sauté about half a minute. Pour egg mixture into skillet. Stir and fold gently until cream cheese is melted and eggs are cooked to your liking. Serve immediately.

Breakfast Strata

Makes 8 servings • Each serving: 16 grams protein • 22 grams carbohydrate
To reduce carbohydrates, use a low-carbohydrate bread.

3 tablespoons softened unsalted
butter

8 slices whole-grain bread, crusts
removed

1 cup sliced brown or white
mushrooms

1 cup artichoke hearts, canned in
water, drained and chopped

1 tablespoon chopped fresh parsley

½ pound grated mozzarella cheese

8 eggs

1 cup all-dairy heavy cream

¾ cup water

1 tablespoon Dijon mustard

freshly ground black pepper,
to taste

Butter both sides of bread and arrange on bottom of a greased
9 x 13-inch baking pan, cutting bread if necessary to fit snugly inside
pan. Sprinkle mushrooms, artichoke hearts and parsley over bread.
Top with grated cheese.

In a small bowl, using a fork, beat eggs with cream, water, mustard
and black pepper. Pour egg mixture over bread. Cover and chill several hours or overnight. Bring to room temperature. Preheat oven to
350°. Bake strata 1 hour. Let sit 5 minutes before slicing.

Breakfast Tacos

Makes 4 servings • Each serving: 20 grams protein • 17 grams carbohydrate
(Nutritional information does not include salsa)

4 strips vegetarian Canadian
  bacon

1 tablespoon unsalted butter

2 tablespoons minced red onion

1 small minced fresh jalapeño
  pepper; or 1 to 2 tablespoons
  canned diced green chilies, to
  taste [wear rubber gloves to
  prepare fresh jalapeño pepper]

4 eggs

freshly ground black pepper,
  to taste

¼ teaspoon dried oregano

½ cup grated Monterey Jack cheese

4 corn tortillas

¼ cup whole sour cream

½ diced ripe avocado

1 tablespoon chopped fresh cilantro

⅓ cup salsa (see Salsas starting
  on page 296), or store-bought

In a nonstick skillet, cook vegetarian Canadian bacon over medium-high heat until crisp. Remove from pan and dice. Set aside.

In the same skillet, melt butter over medium-high heat. When butter is hot and bubbly, add onion and jalapeño pepper and cook until softened, about 5 minutes.

In a medium bowl, using a fork, whisk eggs, black pepper and oregano until well blended. Pour eggs into skillet with onion and chilies and cook, stirring gently, until eggs begin to set, about 2 minutes. Add diced vegetarian Canadian bacon and grated cheese and cook until eggs are firm. Remove from heat.

Heat tortillas by placing them one at a time over an open flame and turning with tongs until puffed up and softened; or layer tortillas between paper towels and microwave on high for 10 to 20 seconds until heated and puffed up.

Spoon ¼ of prepared mixture in center of each tortilla. Add sour cream, avocado and fresh cilantro. Fold in half. Serve with salsa on the side.

Creamy Eggs Baked in Individual Ramekins, with Variations

Makes 2 servings • Each serving: 19 grams protein • trace carbohydrate

1 tablespoon unsalted butter	*freshly ground black pepper,*
4 eggs	*to taste*
2 tablespoons grated Parmesan cheese	*¼ cup all-dairy heavy cream*

Preheat oven to 325°. Lightly butter two 8-ounce ramekins. Crack 2 eggs into each ramekin, being careful not to break yolks. Sprinkle with Parmesan cheese. Season to taste with black pepper. Pour 2 tablespoons cream over each ramekin.

Place ramekins on a baking sheet. Bake 10 to 20 minutes, or until set to your liking.

Variations

Florentine Eggs: Into 2 buttered ramekins, divide ¾ cup cooked, drained and chopped fresh spinach. Top with eggs, Parmesan cheese, black pepper and cream. Bake as above.

Makes 2 servings • Each serving: 20 grams protein • trace carbohydrate

Denver Eggs: Dice 1 cup cooked vegetarian deli slices (soy ham), or 4 cooked soy sausages. Divide into 2 buttered ramekins. Top with eggs, Parmesan cheese, black pepper and cream. Bake as above.

Makes 2 servings • Each serving of soy ham: 34 grams protein • trace carbohydrate
Each serving of soy sausage: 31 grams protein • trace carbohydrate

Mushroom Eggs: Sauté 2 cups of sliced brown or white mushrooms in 2 tablespoons unsalted butter. Add ½ teaspoon dried thyme. Drain excess liquid and divide into 2 buttered ramekins. Top with eggs, Parmesan cheese, black pepper and cream. Bake as above.

Makes 2 servings • Each serving: 20 grams protein • trace carbohydrate

Crustless Quiche, with Variations

Makes 6 servings • Each serving: 10 grams protein • trace carbohydrate

4 eggs

1 cup all-dairy heavy cream

½ cup water

*freshly ground black pepper,
    to taste*

dash cayenne pepper

*1 cup grated Gruyère, mozzarella
    or Monterey Jack cheese*

Preheat oven to 350°. In a medium bowl, using a fork, whisk eggs, cream, water, black pepper and cayenne pepper until well blended. Add grated cheese and mix well.

Butter a 9- or 10-inch pie pan. Pour in egg and cheese mixture. Place pie pan on a baking sheet and bake 45 to 50 minutes, or until a knife inserted into center comes out clean. Let cool 5 minutes before slicing.

Variations

Bell Pepper, Mushrooms and Artichoke Hearts: Sauté 2 cups diced red bell peppers and 2 cups sliced brown or white mushrooms in 2 tablespoons unsalted butter. Add 1 cup chopped artichoke hearts and 1 tablespoon fresh slivered basil. Drain excess liquid. Butter a 9- or 10-inch pie pan. Put sautéed vegetables in bottom of pan. Cover with egg and cheese mixture and bake as above.

Makes 6 servings • Each serving: 11 grams protein • 4 grams carbohydrate

Spinach, Olives and Chili: Combine 1 cup cooked, drained and chopped fresh spinach, ⅓ cup diced green olives, 1 tablespoon diced green chilies and 2 teaspoons dried oregano. Butter a 9- or 10-inch pie pan. Put sautéed vegetables in bottom of pan. Cover with egg and cheese mixture and bake as above.

Makes 6 servings • Each serving: 11 grams protein • trace carbohydrate

Mixed Mushrooms: Sauté 2 cups mixed mushrooms (shitake, oyster, white or brown cremini) and 1 teaspoon dried thyme in 2 tablespoons unsalted butter. Drain excess liquid. Butter a 9- or 10-inch pie pan. Put sautéed vegetables in bottom of pan. Cover with egg and cheese mixture and bake as above. Remove from oven and sprinkle with 2 tablespoons grated Parmesan cheese.

Makes 6 servings • Each serving: 11 grams protein • trace carbohydrate

Broccoli, Scallion and Cheese: Combine 1 cup steamed chopped broccoli florets and ½ cup minced scallions. Butter a 9- or 10-inch pie pan. Put sautéed vegetables in bottom of pan. Cover with egg and cheese mixture and bake as above. Remove from oven and sprinkle with chopped parsley.

Makes 6 servings • Each serving: 11 grams protein • trace carbohydrate

Eggs Florentine

Makes 4 servings • Each serving: 23 grams protein • 13 grams carbohydrate
To reduce carbohydrates use a low-carbohydrate bread instead of English muffin.

*2 bunches spinach equal to about
2 cups cooked spinach, well
drained and chopped; or
16 ounces packaged frozen
spinach, thawed, drained
and chopped*

1 tablespoon white vinegar

8 eggs

*2 whole-grain English muffins
cut in halves*

*Classic Blender
Hollandaise Sauce
(see recipe, page 302)*

Wash spinach well, removing stems. With water still clinging to leaves, place in a medium saucepan with a tight-fitting lid. Turn heat to medium-high and steam until leaves are wilted, about 2 to 3 minutes. Drain in a colander, pressing out all liquid with the back of a wooden spoon. Chop and set aside.

In a large deep skillet, bring 2 inches of water and vinegar to a boil over high heat. Reduce heat to a simmer. Crack eggs, one at a time, into a small bowl and tip gently into boiling water. Repeat with all eggs. Cover skillet and cook 3 minutes for soft yolks, 5 minutes for firmer yolks. Using a slotted spoon, remove eggs from water and drain thoroughly.

Toast English muffins. Arrange spinach on top of muffins, followed by poached eggs. Top with Classic Blender Hollandaise Sauce (see recipe, page 302).

Greek Eggs

Makes 2 servings • Each serving: 28 grams protein • 3 grams carbohydrate

*1 bunch spinach equal to about
1 cup cooked spinach, well
drained and chopped; or 8
ounces packaged frozen spinach,
thawed, drained and chopped*

4 eggs

*1 tablespoon all-dairy heavy
cream*

*freshly ground black pepper,
to taste*

1½ tablespoons unsalted butter

2 tablespoons chopped red onion

1 minced garlic clove

2 teaspoons dried oregano

½ cup crumbled feta cheese

Wash spinach well, removing stems. With water still clinging to leaves, place in a medium saucepan with a tight-fitting lid. Turn heat to medium-high and steam until leaves are wilted, about 2 to 3 minutes. Drain in a colander, pressing out all liquid with the back of a wooden spoon. Chop coarsely and set aside.

In a medium bowl, using a fork, whisk eggs, cream and black pepper. In a 10-inch nonstick skillet, melt butter over medium-high heat. When butter is hot and bubbly, add onion and garlic and cook until softened, about 5 minutes. Add spinach, oregano and egg mixture. Reduce heat to medium. Cook, stirring slowly, folding eggs gently toward center of pan until cooked to your liking. Stir in feta cheese and cook until heated through. Serve immediately.

Huevos Rancheros

Makes 4 servings • Each serving: 28 grams protein • 27 grams carbohydrate
(Nutritional information does not include salsa)

Ranchero Sauce

1 tablespoon pure-pressed
  extra virgin olive oil

½ cup chopped red onion

1 minced garlic clove

½ cup canned red enchilada
  sauce

½ cup Basic Tomato Sauce
  (see recipe, page 300), or
  store-bought, or ½ cup
  chopped fresh tomatoes

½ teaspoon dried oregano

1 teaspoon chili powder

¼ teaspoon ground cumin

freshly ground black pepper,
  to taste

2 tablespoons chopped fresh
  cilantro

8 eggs

4 corn tortillas

1 cup grated Monterey Jack
  cheese

Topping

1 sliced ripe avocado

⅓ cup whole sour cream

4 sprigs fresh cilantro

½ cup salsa (see Salsas starting
  on page 296), or store-bought

In a medium saucepan, heat oil over medium-high heat. When oil is hot, add onion and garlic and cook until softened, about 5 minutes. Add enchilada sauce, tomato sauce or tomatoes, oregano, chili powder, cumin and black pepper. Mix well. Simmer, uncovered, 10 minutes, stirring occasionally. Add chopped cilantro.

Cook eggs over-easy.

Dip tortillas into heated ranchero sauce briefly to soften and warm. Remove from sauce and put on plates. Top with cooked eggs. Add a layer of cheese, followed by more ranchero sauce which will melt the cheese.

Add avocado slices, sour cream and cilantro sprigs. Serve with salsa on the side.

Oatmeal with Butter and Cream

Makes 2 servings • Each serving: 6 grams protein • 27 grams carbohydrate

Because oatmeal is high in carbohydrates, eat it as a side dish, along with a protein (eggs for example), as part of a balanced meal.

1¾ cups water
1 cup oats
2 tablespoons unsalted butter

2 tablespoons all-dairy heavy cream

In a small saucepan, bring water to a boil. Stir in oats and simmer over low heat 3 to 5 minutes, stirring occasionally. Cover pan, remove from heat and let stand until thickened, about 2 minutes. Use more water for a thinner oatmeal. Serve with butter and cream.

Poached Eggs au Gratin

Makes 2 servings • Each serving: 19 grams protein • trace carbohydrate

1 tablespoon white vinegar
4 eggs
2 tablespoons grated Parmesan cheese

2 teaspoons chopped fresh parsley

In a deep medium skillet, bring 2 inches of water and vinegar to a boil over high heat. Reduce heat to simmer. Crack an egg into a small bowl and tip gently into boiling water. Repeat with all eggs. Cover skillet and cook 3 minutes for soft yolks, 5 minutes for firmer yolks. Using a slotted spoon, remove eggs from water and drain thoroughly. Sprinkle with grated Parmesan cheese and fresh parsley. Serve immediately.

Soy Sausage and Eggs Over-Easy

Makes 2 servings • Each serving: 28 grams protein • trace carbohydrate

1 tablespoon pure-pressed extra
  virgin olive oil

4 soy sausages

1½ tablespoons unsalted butter

4 eggs

freshly ground black pepper,
  to taste

In a medium nonstick skillet, heat oil over medium-high heat. When oil is hot, add soy sausages and cook, turning occasionally, until well browned. Remove from pan and set aside.

In a clean medium nonstick skillet, melt butter over medium-high heat. When butter is hot and bubbly, crack eggs into pan. Cook 2 to 3 minutes until whites are firm and yolks are still soft. Using a spatula, flip eggs and continue cooking another 30 seconds, or until yolks are set to your liking. Season to taste with black pepper.

Vegetarian Canadian Bacon and Eggs

Makes 2 servings • Each serving: 32 grams protein • trace carbohydrate

6 slices vegetarian Canadian
  bacon

1½ tablespoons unsalted butter

4 eggs

freshly ground black pepper,
  to taste

In a medium nonstick skillet, cook vegetarian Canadian bacon over medium-high heat until crisp.

In a clean skillet, melt butter over medium-high heat. When butter is hot and bubbly, crack eggs into pan. Cook 2 to 3 minutes until whites are firm and yolks are cooked to your liking. Season to taste with black pepper.

Frittatas and Fabulous Variations

Frittatas are best known in Italy. These open-faced omelets are cooked in a flameproof skillet, then placed briefly under a broiler to puff up and brown.

Basic Frittata

Makes 2 servings • Each serving: 24 grams protein • trace carbohydrate

4 eggs

2 tablespoons all-dairy heavy cream

2 teaspoons minced fresh herbs (parsley, thyme, basil, oregano, dill)

freshly ground black pepper, to taste

dash cayenne pepper

2 tablespoons unsalted butter

½ cup grated mozzarella cheese

Preheat broiler. In a medium bowl, using a fork, whisk eggs, cream, fresh herbs, black pepper and cayenne pepper. Set aside.

In a 10-inch flameproof skillet, melt butter over medium-high heat. When butter is hot and bubbly, add egg mixture. As eggs cook, lift edges to allow uncooked egg to seep underneath. When bottom is set but top is still moist, spread cheese over eggs and place under broiler. Broil 1 to 2 minutes, checking frequently, until top is golden and puffed up.

Avocado and Cream Cheese Frittata

Makes 2 servings • Each serving: 22 grams protein • 9 grams carbohydrate

4 eggs

2 tablespoons all-dairy heavy
   cream

freshly ground black pepper,
   to taste

dash cayenne pepper

1 tablespoon unsalted butter

Filling

1 small diced red onion

1 minced garlic clove

1½ tablespoons unsalted butter

3 tablespoons cream cheese, cut
   into small cubes

1 sliced ripe avocado, for topping

Preheat broiler. In a medium bowl, using a fork, whisk eggs, cream, black pepper and cayenne pepper. Set aside.

In a nonstick skillet, melt 1 tablespoon butter over medium-high heat. When butter is hot and bubbly, add onion and garlic and sauté until softened, about 5 minutes. Set aside.

In a 10-inch flameproof skillet, melt 1½ tablespoons butter over medium-high heat. When butter is hot and bubbly, add egg mixture. As eggs cook, lift edges to allow uncooked egg to seep underneath. When bottom is set but top is still moist, place cream-cheese cubes and onion mixture over eggs and place under broiler. Broil 1 to 2 minutes, checking frequently, until top is golden and puffed up. Top with sliced avocado.

Cottage Cheesy Frittata

Makes 2 servings • Each serving: 28 grams protein • 2 grams carbohydrate

4 eggs

2 tablespoons all-dairy heavy
cream

freshly ground black pepper,
to taste

dash cayenne pepper

Filling

1 bunch spinach equal to about
1 cup cooked spinach, well
drained and chopped; or
8 ounces packaged frozen
spinach, thawed, drained and
chopped

½ cup whole cottage cheese

2 tablespoons grated Parmesan
cheese

2 tablespoons slivered fresh basil,
or 2 teaspoons dried basil

2 tablespoons unsalted butter

Preheat broiler. In a medium bowl, using a fork, whisk eggs, cream, black pepper and cayenne pepper. Set aside.

Wash spinach well, removing stems. With water still clinging to leaves, place in medium saucepan with tight-fitting lid. Turn heat to medium-high and steam until leaves are wilted, about 2 to 3 minutes. Drain in a colander, pressing out all liquid with the back of a wooden spoon. Chop.

In a small bowl combine cottage cheese, Parmesan cheese, spinach and basil. Mix well with a fork until blended. Set aside.

In a 10-inch flameproof skillet, melt butter over medium-high heat. When butter is hot and bubbly, add egg mixture. As eggs cook, lift edges to allow uncooked egg to seep underneath. When bottom is set but top is still moist, spread filling over eggs and place under broiler. Broil 1 to 2 minutes, checking frequently, until top is golden and puffed up.

Mushroom and Artichoke Hearts Frittata

Makes 2 servings • Each serving: 22 grams protein • 5 grams carbohydrate

4 eggs

2 tablespoons all-dairy heavy cream

freshly ground black pepper, to taste

dash cayenne pepper

Filling

2 tablespoons unsalted butter

2 cups sliced brown or white mushrooms

½ cup artichoke hearts, canned in water, drained and chopped

1 teaspoon minced fresh rosemary, or any other fresh herb

2 tablespoons unsalted butter

2 tablespoons grated Parmesan cheese

Preheat broiler. In a medium bowl, using a fork, whisk eggs, cream, black pepper and cayenne pepper. Set aside.

In a 10-inch flameproof skillet, melt 2 tablespoons butter over medium-high heat. When butter is hot and bubbly, add mushrooms and sauté until softened, about 5 minutes. Add artichoke hearts and herbs and cook until heated through. Drain excess liquid and set aside.

In the same pan, melt 2 tablespoons butter over medium-high heat. When butter is hot and bubbly, add egg mixture. As eggs cook, lift edges to allow uncooked egg to seep underneath. When bottom is set but top is still moist, spread filling over eggs. Sprinkle with Parmesan cheese and place under broiler. Broil 1 to 2 minutes, checking frequently, until top is golden and puffed up.

Roasted Pepper and Chèvre (Goat Cheese) Frittata

Makes 2 servings • Each serving: 22 grams protein • 2 grams carbohydrate

4 eggs

2 tablespoons all-dairy heavy cream

freshly ground black pepper, to taste

dash cayenne pepper

Filling

1 red bell pepper, or ¼ cup store-bought roasted red bell peppers

2 ounces fresh chèvre (goat cheese), crumbled

1 tablespoon slivered fresh basil, or 1 teaspoon dried basil

2 tablespoons chopped raw pecans

1 teaspoon grated lemon zest

2 tablespoons unsalted butter

Preheat broiler. In a medium bowl, using a fork, whisk eggs, cream, black pepper and cayenne pepper. Set aside.

If using a fresh bell pepper, roast whole pepper directly over a gas flame or under preheated broiler on a broiler rack. Using tongs, turn pepper frequently until blistered and blackened on all sides. Place pepper in a bowl with a plate on top. Let steam for 15 minutes to loosen skins. Peel off all charred skin. Discard skin and seeds. Cut roasted flesh into slivers.

In a small bowl, combine slivered red bell pepper, goat cheese, basil, pecans and lemon zest. Set aside.

In a 10-inch flameproof skillet, melt butter over medium-high heat. When butter is hot and bubbly, add egg mixture. As eggs cook, lift edges to allow uncooked egg to seep underneath. When bottom is set but top is still moist, spread chèvre filling over egg mixture and place under broiler. Broil 1 to 2 minutes, checking frequently, until top is golden and puffed up.

Soy Sausage, Onion and Cheese Frittata

Makes 2 servings • Each serving: 33 grams protein • trace carbohydrate

4 eggs

2 tablespoons all-dairy heavy cream

freshly ground black pepper, to taste

dash cayenne pepper

2 tablespoons unsalted butter

Filling

1 tablespoon pure-pressed extra virgin olive oil

3 thinly sliced soy sausages

1 tablespoon unsalted butter

½ cup diced onion

2 teaspoons chopped fresh rosemary, or ½ teaspoon dried rosemary

½ cup grated mozzarella cheese

Preheat broiler. In a medium bowl, using a fork, whisk eggs, cream, black pepper and cayenne pepper. Set aside.

In a 10-inch flameproof skillet, heat oil over medium-high heat. When oil is hot, add sausage slices and cook until well browned. Remove from pan and set aside. In same skillet, melt 1 tablespoon butter. When butter is hot and bubbly, add onion and sauté until softened, about 5 minutes. Add cooked sausage and rosemary, and mix well. Remove from pan and set aside.

In the same pan, melt 2 tablespoons butter over medium-high heat. When butter is hot and bubbly, add egg mixture. As eggs cook, lift edges to allow uncooked egg to seep underneath. When bottom is set but top is still moist, spread sausage filling over eggs. Sprinkle top with grated mozzarella cheese and place under broiler. Broil 1 to 2 minutes, checking frequently, until top is golden and puffed up.

Spanish-Style Tortilla Española Frittata

Makes 2 servings • Each serving: 21 grams protein • 26 grams carbohydrate

4 eggs

2 tablespoons all-dairy heavy
   cream

freshly ground black pepper,
   to taste

dash cayenne pepper

2 tablespoons unsalted butter

Filling

2 tablespoons pure-pressed extra
   virgin olive oil

½ cup diced onion

1 minced garlic clove

1 large cooked and diced baking
   potato (peeled, if desired)

2 tablespoons grated Parmesan
   cheese

1 tablespoon minced fresh
   parsley, for garnish

paprika, for garnish

Preheat broiler. In a medium bowl, using a fork, whisk eggs, cream, black pepper and cayenne pepper. Set aside.

In a 10-inch flameproof skillet, heat oil over medium-high heat. When oil is hot, add onion and garlic and sauté until softened, about 5 minutes. Add potato and stir until heated through. Remove from pan and set aside.

In the same pan, melt butter over medium-high heat. When butter is hot and bubbly, add egg mixture. As eggs cook, lift edges to allow uncooked egg to seep underneath. When bottom is set but top is still moist, spread potato filling over eggs. Sprinkle top with Parmesan cheese and place under broiler. Broil 1 to 2 minutes, checking frequently, until top is golden and puffed up. Sprinkle with parsley and paprika.

Spicy Tofu Frittata

Makes 2 servings • Each serving: 26 grams protein • trace carbohydrate

4 eggs

2 tablespoons all-dairy heavy cream

freshly ground black pepper, to taste

dash cayenne pepper

2 tablespoons unsalted butter

Filling

2 tablespoons unsalted butter

½ cup diced red bell peppers

¼ cup diced red onion

½ cup diced green olives

½ cup cubed firm tofu, drained and pressed (for directions, see "All You Need to Know About Tofu," page 10)

¼ to ½ teaspoon red-pepper flakes, to taste

1 tablespoon grated Parmesan cheese

finely chopped fresh parsley, or cilantro, for garnish

Preheat broiler. In a medium bowl, using a fork, whisk eggs, cream, black pepper and cayenne pepper. Set aside.

In a 10-inch flameproof skillet, melt 2 tablespoons butter over medium-high heat. When butter is hot and bubbly, add bell peppers and onion and sauté until softened, about 5 minutes. Add green olives, tofu and red-pepper flakes and stir until heated through. Remove from pan and set aside.

In the same pan, melt 2 tablespoons butter over medium-high heat. When butter is hot and bubbly, add egg mixture. As eggs cook, lift edges to allow uncooked egg to seep underneath. When bottom is set but top is still moist, spread filling over eggs. Sprinkle top with Parmesan cheese and place under broiler. Broil 1 to 2 minutes, checking frequently, until top is golden and puffed up. Sprinkle with parsley or cilantro.

Omelets

Cream Cheese and Avocado Omelet

Makes 2 servings • Each serving: 22 grams protein • 12 grams carbohydrate

4 eggs

2 tablespoons all-dairy heavy cream

freshly ground black pepper, to taste

3 ounces cream cheese, cut into ½-inch cubes

2 tablespoons unsalted butter

Filling

1 diced ripe avocado

1 small diced tomato

1 tablespoon minced fresh chives; or 1 tablespoon finely chopped scallions

In a medium bowl, using a fork, whisk eggs, cream and black pepper. Add cream-cheese cubes and mix well. In a 10-inch nonstick skillet, melt butter over medium-high heat. When butter is hot and bubbly, add egg mixture, reduce heat to medium and cook, lifting edges to allow uncooked egg to seep underneath.

In a medium bowl, combine avocado, tomato and chives or scallions. When bottom layer of egg is cooked but top is still moist, spread avocado filling over one side of omelet. Gently fold omelet in half. Cook half a minute longer. Slide omelet onto a plate and serve immediately.

Curried Tofu Omelet

Makes 2 servings • Each serving: 26 grams protein • trace carbohydrate

4 eggs

*2 tablespoons all-dairy heavy
   cream*

*freshly ground black pepper,
   to taste*

dash cayenne pepper

2 tablespoons unsalted butter

Filling

*½ cup crumbled firm tofu,
   drained and pressed (for
   directions, see "All You Need
   to Know About Tofu," page 10)*

¼ cup whole sour cream

1 teaspoon curry powder

*2 tablespoons finely chopped
   scallions*

In a medium bowl, using a fork, whisk eggs, cream and black pepper. Set aside. In a small bowl, combine tofu, sour cream, curry powder and scallions.

In a 10-inch nonstick skillet, melt butter over medium-high heat. When butter is hot and bubbly, add egg mixture, reduce heat to medium and cook, lifting edges to allow uncooked egg to seep underneath. When bottom layer of egg is cooked but top is still moist, spread tofu filling over one side of omelet. Gently fold in half. Cook half a minute longer. Slide omelet onto a plate and serve immediately.

Greek Omelet

Makes 2 servings • Each serving: 28 grams protein • 3 grams carbohydrate

4 eggs

2 tablespoons all-dairy heavy
cream

freshly ground black pepper,
to taste

dash cayenne pepper

2 tablespoons unsalted butter

Filling

1 bunch spinach equal to about
1 cup cooked spinach, well
drained and chopped; or
8 ounces packaged frozen
spinach, thawed, drained and
chopped

1 tablespoon unsalted butter

2 tablespoons chopped red onion

½ cup crumbled feta cheese

2 teaspoons dried oregano

In a medium bowl, using a fork, whisk eggs, cream and black pepper. Set aside.

Wash spinach well, removing stems. With water still clinging to leaves, place in a medium saucepan with a tight-fitting lid. Turn heat to medium-high and steam until leaves are wilted, about 2 to 3 minutes. Drain in a colander, pressing out all liquid with the back of a wooden spoon. Chop fine and set aside.

In a 10-inch nonstick skillet, melt 1 tablespoon butter over medium-high heat. When butter is hot and bubbly, add onion and sauté until softened, about 5 minutes. Remove from pan and set aside.

In a small bowl, combine sautéed onion, feta cheese, spinach and oregano.

In the same pan, melt 2 tablespoons butter over medium-high heat. When butter is hot and bubbly, add egg mixture, reduce heat to medium and cook, lifting edges to allow uncooked egg to seep underneath.

When bottom layer of egg is cooked but top is still moist, spread spinach filling over one side of omelet. Gently fold in half. Cook half a minute longer. Slide omelet onto a plate and serve immediately.

Mushroom and Gorgonzola Omelet with Walnuts

Makes 2 servings • Each serving: 23 grams protein • 3 grams carbohydrate

4 eggs

2 tablespoons all-dairy heavy cream

freshly ground black pepper, to taste

Filling

2 tablespoons unsalted butter

1 cup thinly sliced brown or white mushrooms

¼ cup finely chopped scallions

2 tablespoons crumbled Gorgonzola, or any other blue-veined cheese

2 tablespoons slivered fresh basil, or 2 teaspoons dried basil

¼ cup chopped raw walnuts

In a medium bowl, using a fork, whisk eggs, cream and black pepper. Set aside.

In a 10-inch nonstick skillet, melt butter over medium-high heat. When butter is hot and bubbly, add sliced mushrooms and scallions and sauté, stirring occasionally, until softened and most of liquid has evaporated, about 5 minutes.

Add beaten egg mixture to mushrooms and scallions and cook over medium heat until eggs begin to set. Lift edges to allow uncooked egg to seep underneath. When bottom layer of egg is cooked but top is still moist, spread crumbled Gorgonzola, basil and walnuts over one side of omelet. Gently fold in half. Cook half a minute longer to melt cheese. Slide omelet onto a plate and serve immediately.

Soy Sausage and Cheese Omelet

Makes 2 servings • Each serving: 32 grams protein • trace carbohydrate

4 eggs

2 tablespoons all-dairy heavy
cream

freshly ground black pepper,
to taste

Filling

2 tablespoons pure-pressed extra
virgin olive oil

½ cup diced onion

1 minced garlic clove

¼ pound diced soy sausage

1 teaspoon dried oregano

2 tablespoons unsalted butter

¼ cup grated Monterey Jack
cheese

In a medium bowl, using a fork, whisk eggs, cream and black pepper.
Set aside.

In a 10-inch nonstick skillet, heat oil over medium-high heat. When
oil is hot, add onion, garlic, soy sausage and oregano and sauté until
sausage is browned. Remove from pan and set aside.

In the same pan, melt butter over medium-high heat. When butter
is hot and bubbly, add egg mixture, reduce heat to medium and cook,
lifting edges to allow uncooked egg to seep underneath.

When bottom layer of egg is cooked but top is still moist, spread
sausage filling and grated cheese over one side of omelet. Gently fold
in half. Cook half a minute longer. Slide omelet onto a plate and serve
immediately.

Spinach and Brie Omelet

Makes 2 servings • Each serving: 31 grams protein • trace carbohydrate

4 eggs

2 tablespoons all-dairy heavy cream

freshly ground black pepper, to taste

Filling

1 bunch spinach equal to about 1 cup cooked spinach, well drained and chopped; or 8 ounces packaged frozen spinach, thawed, drained and chopped

2 tablespoons unsalted butter

2 tablespoons diced red onion

¼ pound finely sliced Brie cheese

1 tablespoon slivered fresh basil, or 1 teaspoon dried basil

In a medium bowl, using a fork, whisk eggs, cream and black pepper. Set aside.

Wash spinach well, removing stems. With water still clinging to leaves, place in a medium saucepan with a tight-fitting lid. Turn heat to medium-high and steam until leaves are wilted, about 2 to 3 minutes. Drain in a colander, pressing out all liquid with the back of a wooden spoon. Chop and set aside.

In a 10-inch nonstick skillet, melt butter over medium-high heat. When butter is hot and bubbly, add onion and cook until softened, about 3 to 5 minutes. Add egg mixture, reduce heat to medium and continue cooking, lifting edges to allow uncooked egg to seep underneath.

When bottom layer of egg is cooked but top is still moist, arrange Brie cheese slices on one side of omelet. Spread cooked spinach over cheese and sprinkle with fresh or dried basil. Gently fold omelet in half. Cook half a minute longer or until cheese melts. Slide omelet onto a plate and serve immediately.

Sun-Dried Tomato and Chèvre (Goat Cheese) Omelet

Makes 2 servings • Each serving: 25 grams protein • 7 grams carbohydrate

4 eggs

2 tablespoons all-dairy heavy cream

freshly ground black pepper, to taste

Filling

¼ cup slivered sun-dried tomatoes, packed in olive oil and drained (reserve oil)

3 tablespoons crumbled chèvre (goat cheese)

2 tablespoons finely slivered fresh basil, or *2 teaspoons dried basil*

3 tablespoons diced green olives

In a medium bowl, using a fork, whisk eggs, cream and black pepper. Set aside.

Combine sun-dried tomatoes with crumbled goat cheese, basil and green olives. Set aside.

In a 10-inch nonstick skillet, pour in 2 tablespoons of drained olive oil from sun-dried tomatoes. When oil is hot, pour in egg mixture. Cook over medium-high heat until eggs begin to set. Lift edges to allow uncooked egg to seep underneath. When bottom layer of egg is cooked but top is still moist, spread sun-dried tomato and cheese mixture over one side of omelet. Gently fold omelet in half. Cook half a minute longer until filling is hot. Slide omelet onto a plate and serve immediately.

Western Omelet

Makes 2 servings.
Each serving made with vegetarian deli slices: 31 grams protein • trace carbohydrate
Each serving made with soy sausages: 28 grams protein • trace carbohydrate

4 eggs

2 tablespoons all-dairy heavy
cream

freshly ground black pepper,
to taste

Filling

2 tablespoons unsalted butter

3 tablespoons diced onion

½ diced green bell pepper

½ cup diced vegetarian deli slices
(soy ham) or soy sausages

1 tablespoon chopped fresh
parsley, for garnish

In a medium bowl, using a fork, whisk eggs, cream and black pepper.
Set aside.

In a 10-inch nonstick skillet, melt butter over medium-high heat.
When butter is hot and bubbly, add onion and bell pepper. Cook until
softened, about 5 minutes. Add vegetarian deli slices or sausage and
cook another 2 minutes.

Add egg mixture, reduce heat to medium and continue cooking, lifting edges to allow uncooked egg to seep underneath. Cook until egg is
set and bottom is lightly browned. Gently fold omelet in half and
sprinkle with parsley. Slide omelet onto a plate and serve immediately.

Scrambled Eggs

Basic Scrambled Eggs

Makes 2 servings • Each serving: 16 grams protein • trace carbohydrate

4 eggs

2 tablespoons all-dairy heavy cream

freshly ground black pepper, to taste

2 tablespoons unsalted butter

In a medium bowl, using a fork, whisk eggs, cream and black pepper. Set aside.

In a 10-inch nonstick skillet, melt butter over medium-high heat. When butter is hot and bubbly, add eggs to pan. Reduce heat to medium. Gently stir egg mixture with a wooden spoon until eggs are soft, creamy and cooked to your liking. Serve immediately.

Asian Scramble

Makes 2 servings • Each serving: 17 grams protein • trace carbohydrate

4 eggs

2 tablespoons all-dairy heavy cream

freshly ground black pepper, to taste

2 tablespoons pure-pressed peanut oil

2 tablespoons minced scallions

2 tablespoons minced fresh cilantro

1 teaspoon peeled and finely minced fresh ginger

¼ cup thinly sliced celery stalks

1 cup sliced brown or white mushrooms

2 teaspoons low-sodium tamari soy sauce

In a small bowl, using a fork, whisk eggs, cream and black pepper. Set aside.

In a 10-inch nonstick skillet, heat oil over medium-high heat. When oil is hot, add scallions, cilantro, ginger, celery, mushrooms and soy sauce and sauté until softened, about 5 minutes. Drain excess liquid from pan. Add eggs to pan. Reduce heat to medium and gently stir egg mixture with a wooden spoon until cooked to your liking. Serve immediately.

Deli Scramble

Makes 2 servings • Each serving: 28 grams protein • trace carbohydrate

4 eggs

2 tablespoons all-dairy heavy cream

freshly ground black pepper, to taste

2 tablespoons unsalted butter

½ cup diced onion

½ cup diced soy sausage

In a small bowl, using a fork, whisk eggs, cream and black pepper. Set aside.

In a 10-inch nonstick skillet, melt butter over medium-high heat. When butter is hot and bubbly, add onion and soy sausage and sauté until sausage is browned.

Add eggs to pan. Reduce heat to medium. Gently stir egg mixture with a wooden spoon until cooked to your liking. Serve immediately.

Santa Barbara Scrambled Eggs

Makes 2 servings • Each serving: 23 grams protein • 3 grams carbohydrate

4 eggs

2 tablespoons all-dairy heavy
  cream

freshly ground black pepper,
  to taste

2 tablespoons unsalted butter

1 cup sliced brown or white
  mushrooms

3 ounces cream cheese, cut into
  ½-inch cubes

2 tablespoons grated Parmesan
  cheese

2 tablespoons slivered fresh basil,
  or 1 teaspoon dried basil

1 tablespoon minced fresh parsley

In a medium bowl, using a fork, whisk eggs, cream and black pepper. Set aside.

In a 10-inch nonstick skillet, melt butter over medium-high heat. When butter is hot and bubbly, add sliced mushrooms. Cook until mushrooms are softened, about 5 minutes. Drain excess liquid.

Pour beaten egg mixture over mushrooms. Reduce heat to medium. Gently stir egg mixture with a wooden spoon, about 1 minute. Sprinkle cream cheese, Parmesan cheese, basil and parsley evenly over eggs. Continue folding until cheese is melted and eggs are set. Serve immediately.

South of the Border Scramble

Makes 2 servings • Each serving: 21 grams protein • 19 grams carbohydrate

4 eggs

2 tablespoons all-dairy heavy
  cream

freshly ground black pepper,
  to taste

2 tablespoons unsalted butter

½ diced red onion

½ diced bell pepper

1 small diced fresh jalapeño
  pepper; or 1 to 2 tablespoons
  canned diced green chilies, to
  taste [wear rubber gloves to
  prepare fresh jalapeño pepper]

½ cup corn

1 diced medium tomato

2 tablespoons chopped fresh
  cilantro

Topping

1 sliced ripe avocado

2 tablespoons whole sour cream

2 sprigs fresh cilantro

In a small bowl, using a fork, whisk eggs, cream and black pepper. Set aside.

In a 10-inch nonstick skillet, melt butter over medium-high heat. When butter is hot and bubbly, add onion, bell pepper and jalapeño pepper and sauté until softened, about 5 minutes. Add corn, tomato, cilantro and egg mixture. Gently stir egg mixture with a wooden spoon until cooked to your liking. Arrange eggs on a plate and top with avocado, sour cream and cilantro sprigs. Serve immediately.

Vegetarian Canadian Bacon Scramble

Makes 2 servings • Each serving: 34 grams protein • trace carbohydrate

4 slices vegetarian Canadian
  bacon

4 eggs

2 tablespoons all-dairy heavy
  cream

freshly ground black pepper,
  to taste

2 tablespoons unsalted butter

1 diced medium tomato

½ cup grated mozzarella cheese

In a medium nonstick skillet, cook vegetarian Canadian bacon over medium-high heat until crisp. Dice and set aside.

In a small bowl, using a fork, whisk eggs, cream and black pepper. Set aside.

In a 10-inch nonstick skillet, melt butter over medium-high heat. When butter is hot and bubbly, add egg mixture to pan. Reduce heat to medium. Add diced vegetarian Canadian bacon, tomato and grated cheese. Gently move egg mixture around with a wooden spoon until cooked to your liking and cheese is melted. Serve immediately.

Scrambled Tofu

Basic Scrambled Tofu

Makes 2 servings • Each serving: 23 grams protein • trace carbohydrate

2 tablespoons unsalted butter

⅔ pound firm tofu, drained, pressed and crumbled (for directions, see "All You Need to Know About Tofu," page 10)

freshly ground black pepper, to taste

In a 10-inch nonstick skillet, melt butter over medium-high heat. When butter is hot and bubbly, add crumbled tofu and sauté until lightly browned and heated through, gently stirring tofu mixture with a wooden spoon. Season to taste with black pepper. Serve hot.

Curried Tofu Scramble

Makes 2 servings • Each serving: 24 grams protein • 7 grams carbohydrate

2 tablespoons unsalted butter

⅔ pound firm tofu, drained, pressed and crumbled (for directions, see "All You Need to Know About Tofu," page 10)

freshly ground black pepper, to taste

1 teaspoon curry powder

2 tablespoons Apricot and Raisin Chutney, (see recipe, page 287), or store-bought chutney (no sugar added)

¼ cup minced scallions

2 teaspoons minced fresh cilantro

2 teaspoons fresh lime juice

In a 10-inch nonstick skillet, melt butter over medium-high heat. When butter is hot and bubbly, add crumbled tofu, black pepper, curry powder, chutney, scallions and cilantro. Sauté until lightly browned and heated through, gently stirring tofu mixture with a wooden spoon. Sprinkle with lime juice and serve hot.

Fiesta Tofu Scramble

Makes 2 servings • Each serving: 31 grams protein • 26 grams carbohydrate

2 tablespoons pure-pressed
  monounsaturated vegetable oil

1 large diced potato (peeled,
  if desired)

¼ diced red onion

1 minced garlic clove

⅔ pound firm tofu, drained,
  pressed and crumbled (for
  directions, see "All You Need to
  Know About Tofu," page 10)

freshly ground black pepper,
  to taste

¼ cup grated Parmesan cheese

¼ cup canned diced green chilies

¼ to ½ teaspoon red-pepper
  flakes, to taste

2 tablespoons minced fresh
  cilantro

In a 10-inch nonstick skillet, heat oil over medium-high heat. When oil is hot, add potato, onion and garlic. Sauté until potato is cooked through about 8 minutes, stirring often. Add tofu, black pepper, Parmesan cheese, chilies, red-pepper flakes and cilantro. Sauté until lightly browned and heated through, gently stirring tofu mixture with a wooden spoon. Serve hot.

Greek Tofu Scramble

Makes 2 servings • Each serving: 31 grams protein • 2 grams carbohydrate

*1 bunch spinach equal to about
1 cup cooked spinach, well
drained and chopped; or
8 ounces packaged frozen
spinach, thawed, drained and
chopped*

2 tablespoons unsalted butter

*⅔ pound firm tofu, drained,
pressed and crumbled (for
directions, see "All You Need to
Know About Tofu," page 10)*

*freshly ground black pepper,
to taste*

⅓ cup crumbled feta cheese

¼ cup diced Kalamata olives

2 teaspoons dried oregano

Wash spinach well, removing stems. With water still clinging to leaves, place in a medium saucepan with a tight-fitting lid. Turn heat to medium-high and steam until leaves are wilted, about 2 to 3 minutes. Drain in a colander, pressing out all liquid with the back of a wooden spoon. Chop fine and set aside.

In a 10-inch nonstick skillet, melt butter over medium-high heat. When butter is hot and bubbly, add tofu, black pepper, feta cheese, spinach, olives and oregano. Sauté until heated through, gently stirring tofu mixture with a wooden spoon. Serve hot.

Mushroom-Avocado Tofu Scramble

Makes 2 servings • Each serving: 27 grams protein • 11 grams carbohydrate

2 tablespoons unsalted butter

¼ cup diced onion

1 minced garlic clove

2 cups sliced brown or white
mushrooms

2 small diced zucchini

⅔ pound firm tofu, drained,
pressed and crumbled (for
directions, see "All You Need to
Know About Tofu," page 10)

freshly ground black pepper,
to taste

2 tablespoons slivered fresh basil,
or 2 teaspoons dried basil

1 diced ripe avocado, for garnish

In a 10-inch nonstick skillet, melt butter over medium-high heat.
When butter is hot and bubbly, add onion, garlic, mushrooms and
zucchini. Sauté until softened, about 5 minutes, stirring often. Add
tofu, black pepper, and basil, and sauté until heated through, gently
stirring tofu mixture with a wooden spoon. Garnish with diced avocado and serve hot.

Pesto Tofu Scramble

Makes 2 servings • Each serving: 31 grams protein • 5 grams carbohydrate

2 tablespoons unsalted butter

2 cups sliced brown or white
mushrooms

1 medium diced zucchini

⅔ pound firm tofu, drained,
pressed and crumbled (for
directions, see "All You Need to
Know About Tofu," page 10)

freshly ground black pepper,
to taste

¼ cup Basil Pesto (see recipe,
page 294), or store-bought

In a 10-inch nonstick skillet, melt butter over medium-high heat. When butter is hot and bubbly, add mushrooms and zucchini and sauté until softened, about 5 minutes. Drain excess liquid from pan. Add tofu, black pepper and pesto. Sauté until heated through, gently stirring tofu mixture with a wooden spoon. Serve hot.

Soy Sausage Tofu Scramble

Makes 2 servings • Each serving: 42 grams protein • trace carbohydrate

2 tablespoons pure-pressed extra
  virgin olive oil

4 diced soy sausages

⅔ pound firm tofu, drained,
  pressed and crumbled (for
  directions, see "All You Need to
  Know About Tofu," page 10)

freshly ground black pepper,
  to taste

1 teaspoon dried thyme

½ cup grated mozzarella cheese

In a 10-inch nonstick skillet, heat oil over medium-high heat. When oil is hot, add soy sausages and sauté until browned. Add tofu, black pepper and thyme, and sauté until heated through, gently stirring tofu mixture with a wooden spoon. Add mozzarella cheese and cook until melted. Serve hot.

Sun-Dried Tomato, Chèvre (Goat Cheese) and Tofu Scramble

Makes 2 servings • Each serving: 35 grams protein • 9 grams carbohydrate

2 tablespoons pure-pressed extra virgin olive oil or oil from sun-dried tomatoes

⅔ pound firm tofu, drained, pressed and crumbled (for directions, see "All You Need to Know About Tofu," page 10)

freshly ground black pepper, to taste

2 tablespoons slivered fresh basil, or 2 teaspoons dried basil

⅓ cup slivered sun-dried tomatoes, packed in oil and drained (reserve oil)

½ cup crumbled chèvre (goat cheese)

In a 10-inch nonstick skillet, heat olive oil or drained sun-dried tomato oil over medium-high heat. When oil is hot, add tofu, black pepper, basil and sun-dried tomatoes, and sauté until heated through. Add chèvre (goat cheese) and cook until melted. Serve hot.

Smoothies

If a recipe is high in carbohydrates, it should not be eaten alone as a meal. Instead, combine it with a higher-protein recipe to create a balanced meal.

Peanut Butter Smoothie with Yogurt and Banana

Makes 1 smoothie • 13 grams protein • 28 grams carbohydrate

½ cup whole plain yogurt

2 tablespoons organic peanut butter, chunky or smooth (no honey or sugar added)

½ banana

2 crushed ice cubes

Combine all ingredients in a blender. Blend on high until smooth and creamy.

Peanut Butter Smoothie
with Yogurt and Dates

Makes 1 smoothie • 13 grams protein • 29 grams carbohydrate

½ cup whole plain yogurt

2 tablespoons organic peanut
butter, chunky or smooth
(no honey or sugar added)

2 pitted dates

2 crushed ice cubes

Combine all ingredients in a blender. Blend on high until smooth
and creamy.

Yogurt Smoothie
with Cottage Cheese and Strawberries

Makes 1 smoothie • 12 grams protein • 13 grams carbohydrate

½ cup whole plain yogurt

¼ cup whole cottage cheese

4 strawberries, sliced

2 crushed ice cubes

Combine all ingredients in a blender. Blend on high until smooth
and creamy.

Appetizers, Snacks, Dips and Spreads

Assorted Appetizers and Snacks

Dips

Spreads

Assorted Appetizers and Snacks

Artichokes with Hollandaise Sauce

Makes 4 servings • Each serving: 6 grams protein • 13 grams carbohydrate

4 artichokes

1 quartered lemon

Classic Blender Hollandaise Sauce

With a sharp knife, slice off top of each artichoke and trim stems so that they sit upright. Use kitchen shears to trim points off ends of leaves. Place artichokes in 4 inches of boiling water along with a quartered lemon. Boil uncovered, about 35 to 45 minutes, or until leaves pull away easily and are tender.

Serve with Classic Blender Hollandaise Sauce on the side, in dipping bowls.

Classic Blender Hollandaise Sauce

3 egg yolks*

2 tablespoons fresh lemon juice

dash cayenne pepper

4 ounces (1 stick) unsalted butter melted and bubbling hot

In a blender, combine egg yolks, lemon juice and cayenne pepper, on high for 3 seconds. Remove lid and, with motor running, slowly pour hot butter in a steady stream over eggs. When butter is all poured in, blend an additional 5 seconds. Taste, and adjust seasonings. Serve immediately, or keep sauce warm by placing blender in a bowl of warm water.

Makes about 1 cup.

---

*If you are concerned about using raw eggs, choose an alternate recipe.

Asparagus Spears in Garlic Vinaigrette

Makes 4 servings • Each serving: trace protein • trace carbohydrate

1 pound asparagus, tough ends trimmed

Garlic Vinaigrette

2 tablespoons balsamic vinegar

2 minced garlic cloves

1 teaspoon Dijon mustard

*freshly ground black pepper,
   to taste*

*⅓ cup pure-pressed extra virgin
   olive oil*

*1 tablespoon grated Parmesan
   cheese*

In a large skillet, bring 1 inch of water to a boil over medium-high heat. Add asparagus and cook until tender, about 3 to 6 minutes. Remove from pan, drain and arrange on a serving platter.

In a blender or food processor, blend all vinaigrette ingredients until smooth; or place ingredients in a jar with a tight-fitting lid and shake vigorously until well blended. Pour over asparagus and serve at room temperature.

Cheesy Quesadillas

Makes 8 servings • Each serving: 15 grams protein • 20 grams carbohydrate
(Nutritional information does not include salsa)

Filling

2 tablespoons canned diced green
   chilies

2 cups diced baked marinated
   tofu

¼ cup minced scallions

2 tablespoons minced fresh
   cilantro

1½ cups grated Monterey Jack
   cheese

1 tablespoon pure-pressed
   monounsaturated vegetable oil
   or unsalted butter

8 corn tortillas

Toppings

2 thinly sliced ripe avocados

1 cup whole sour cream

½ cup Papaya or Mango Salsa
(see recipe, page 297)

In a medium bowl, combine filling ingredients.

In a medium nonstick skillet, heat oil or butter over medium-high
heat. When hot, add a corn tortilla and heat on one side before flipping over. Spoon ¼ cup of filling on half of tortilla. Do not overfill.
Fold plain half of tortilla over.

Cook each side about 2 to 3 minutes, until cheese is melted and filling is hot. Add more oil or butter to pan as needed and cook remaining tortillas the same way. Add sliced avocado and sour cream before
serving. Serve salsa on the side.

Curried Deviled Eggs

Makes 12 halves • Each half: 4 grams protein • trace carbohydrate

6 hard-boiled eggs

4 tablespoons mayonnaise
  (made from pure-pressed oil)

2 teaspoons Dijon mustard

1 teaspoon curry powder

cayenne pepper, to taste

2 tablespoons chopped fresh
  cilantro, or parsley, for garnish

paprika, for garnish

To hard boil eggs, place eggs in a saucepan and cover with cold water. Bring to a boil uncovered. Allow to boil for 1 minute, then cover, remove from heat and let sit undisturbed 10 minutes. Rinse eggs under cold water. Crack shells, peel and rinse eggs.

Cut peeled eggs in half lengthwise. Carefully remove yolks and put into a medium bowl. Add remaining ingredients, except cilantro/parsley and paprika. Mash with a fork until smooth. Taste, and adjust seasonings.

Using a small teaspoon, fill egg-white cavities with about 1 tablespoon of curry mixture per egg. Sprinkle tops with cilantro or parsley and paprika. Arrange on a serving platter.

Marinated Mushrooms

Makes 4 servings • Each serving: 2 grams protein • trace carbohydrate

½ pound small brown or white
* mushrooms*

3 tablespoons pure-pressed extra
* virgin olive oil*

1 tablespoon water

juice of 1 lemon

½ teaspoon dried thyme

1 minced garlic clove

4 tablespoons finely chopped
* fresh parsley*

freshly ground black pepper,
* to taste*

Wipe mushrooms clean with a damp cloth. Trim stems and set mushrooms aside.

In a medium saucepan, bring oil, water, lemon juice, thyme, garlic and parsley to a boil. Add mushrooms and simmer 10 minutes, stirring occasionally. Season to taste with black pepper. Put mushrooms into a serving bowl and let cool. Taste, and adjust seasonings. Serve with toothpicks on the side.

Pecan Cheese Ball

Makes 6 servings • Each serving: 9 grams protein • 3 grams carbohydrate

½ cup chopped raw pecans

8 ounces cream cheese, softened at room temperature

4 ounces crumbled Gorgonzola cheese, or *any other blue-veined cheese*

2 tablespoons minced fresh parsley

2 tablespoons slivered fresh basil, or *1 teaspoon dried basil*

freshly ground black pepper, to taste

Put pecans in an ungreased medium skillet, over medium-high heat. Stir nuts or shake pan almost constantly, until pecans are evenly browned and toasted. Remove from pan immediately and set aside to cool.

In a food processor, blend softened cream cheese, Gorgonzola cheese, parsley, basil, black pepper and ¼ cup chopped, toasted pecans until smooth, breaking up any lumps with a spatula.

Form cheese mixture into a ball and place in a small bowl lined with plastic wrap. Seal and refrigerate several hours or overnight. A half hour before serving, remove from refrigerator. Unwrap and sprinkle with ¼ cup reserved pecans. Serve with assorted raw vegetables.

Salad Stix

Makes 8 servings • Each serving: 5 grams protein • 4 grams carbohydrate

16 small fresh mozzarella balls

¼ cup pure-pressed extra virgin olive oil

3 minced garlic cloves

freshly ground black pepper, to taste

2 red bell peppers, roasted and cut into large chunks, or ½ cup store-bought roasted red peppers

16 fresh basil leaves

16 marinated mushrooms, prepared (see recipe, page 69) or store-bought

8 large green olives

2 cups marinated artichoke hearts, drained and cut into chunks

eight 8-inch bamboo skewers

Drain fresh mozzarella balls and rinse with water. In a small bowl mix together oil, garlic and black pepper. Add mozzarella balls and marinate 15 minutes or overnight, if possible.

If using fresh red bell peppers, roast peppers directly over a gas flame, or under preheated broiler on a broiler rack. Using tongs, turn peppers frequently until blistered and blackened on all sides. Place peppers in a bowl with a plate on top. Let steam for 15 minutes to loosen skins. Peel off all charred skin. Discard skin along with seeds. Cut roasted flesh into 1-inch pieces.

Take a bamboo skewer and put on a mozzarella ball moving it down to the base of the stick. Next put on a whole basil leaf followed by a red bell pepper chunk, mushroom, green olive, artichoke heart, basil leaf, red bell pepper chunk, mushroom and mozzarella ball. Repeat with other sticks until all ingredients have been used up.

Arrange on a platter and serve immediately.

Sesame Baked Mushrooms

Makes about 20 mushrooms • Each mushroom: 1 gram protein • 2 grams carbohydrate

¼ cup raw sesame seeds

1 pound medium brown or
   white mushrooms

1 beaten egg

1 teaspoon Dijon mustard

freshly ground black pepper,
   to taste

¼ cup fresh or dried whole-grain
   bread crumbs

Put sesame seeds in an ungreased medium skillet, over medium-high heat. Stir seeds or shake pan almost constantly until seeds are evenly browned and toasted and begin to pop. Remove from pan immediately and set aside.

Preheat oven to 350°. Wipe mushrooms clean with a damp cloth. Trim stems and set mushrooms aside. In a small bowl, using a fork, mix beaten egg with mustard and black pepper. In a separate bowl, mix sesame seeds and bread crumbs.

Spear stem end of mushrooms with a fork. Dip cap into egg mixture, then into bread-crumb mixture. Place on a greased rack with a tinfoil-lined baking sheet underneath. Bake 15 to 20 minutes, until golden brown. Serve hot.

Spicy Mixed Nuts

Makes about 4 cups • Each ¼ cup serving • 6 grams protein • 7 grams carbohydrate

3 tablespoons pure-pressed extra virgin olive oil

2 minced garlic cloves

1 teaspoon low-sodium tamari soy sauce

½ teaspoon ground cumin

1 teaspoon curry powder

dash red-pepper flakes

½ teaspoon chili powder

1 cup whole raw almonds

1 cup whole raw cashews

1 cup raw pecan halves

1 cup whole raw peanuts

Preheat oven to 350°. In a large skillet, heat oil over medium heat. When oil is hot, add garlic and sauté until softened, about 10 seconds. Add soy sauce, cumin, curry powder, red-pepper flakes and chili powder. Stir well. Add mixed nuts and stir until thoroughly coated with spices.

Transfer nut mix to a baking sheet. Bake 15 to 20 minutes, stirring frequently to bake evenly. Remove from oven and cool. Store in an airtight container.

Spinach-and-Cheese-Stuffed Mushrooms

Makes 6 servings • Each serving: 10 grams protein • 3 grams carbohydrate

*1 bunch spinach equal to about
1 cup cooked spinach, well
drained and chopped; or
8 ounces packaged frozen
spinach, thawed, drained and
chopped*

12 large stuffing mushrooms

2 tablespoons unsalted butter

2 tablespoons minced scallions

1 minced garlic clove

*1 cup whole ricotta or whole
cottage cheese*

¼ cup grated Parmesan cheese

*2 tablespoons slivered fresh basil,
or 1 teaspoon dried basil*

*freshly ground black pepper,
to taste*

*2 tablespoons pure-pressed extra
virgin olive oil*

*2 tablespoons grated Parmesan
cheese*

paprika, for garnish

Preheat oven to 375°. Wash spinach well, removing stems. With water still clinging to leaves, place in a medium saucepan with a tight-fitting lid. Turn heat to medium-high and steam until leaves are wilted, about 2 to 3 minutes. Drain in a colander, pressing out all liquid with the back of a wooden spoon. Chop fine and set aside.

Wipe mushrooms clean with a damp cloth. Remove stems and chop fine. Set caps aside. In a small skillet, melt butter over medium-high heat. When butter is hot and bubbly, add scallions, garlic and chopped mushroom stems and sauté until softened, about 5 minutes. Remove from heat and put into a large bowl along with drained spinach, ricotta or cottage cheese, Parmesan cheese, basil and black pepper. Mix well with a wooden spoon. Taste, and adjust seasonings.

Using your fingers, lightly oil tops of mushroom caps. Mound each mushroom cavity with about 1 tablespoon of filling. Arrange mushrooms, cavity-side up, on a greased rack with a tinfoil-lined baking sheet underneath. Sprinkle with Parmesan cheese and paprika. Bake until thoroughly heated, about 15 to 20 minutes. Serve hot.

Dips

Avocado, Cilantro and Gorgonzola Cheese Dip

Makes about 2½ cups • Each ¼ cup serving: 4 grams protein • 4 grams carbohydrate

2 large ripe avocados	3 tablespoons chopped scallions
½ cup crumbled Gorgonzola cheese	2 tablespoons chopped fresh cilantro
1 cup whole sour cream	2 minced garlic cloves
1 tablespoon mayonnaise (made from pure-pressed oil)	dash hot sauce
2 tablespoons fresh lime juice	freshly ground black pepper, to taste

Cut avocados in half. Remove pits and scoop flesh into a medium bowl. Mash coarsely with a fork. Add Gorgonzola cheese, sour cream and mayonnaise and blend well. Add lime juice, scallions, cilantro, garlic, hot sauce and black pepper. Blend until well mixed. Taste, and adjust seasonings. Chill 1 hour before serving.

Mound dip in a small serving bowl and surround with cut-up raw vegetables.

Baba Ganoush

Makes about 2 cups • Each ¼ cup serving: 2 grams protein • trace carbohydrate

2 medium eggplants

2 minced garlic cloves

3 tablespoons sesame tahini

2 to 4 tablespoons fresh lemon
  juice, to taste

½ teaspoon ground cumin

2 tablespoons pure-pressed extra
  virgin olive oil

freshly ground black pepper,
  to taste

dash cayenne pepper

Preheat oven to 425°. Cut eggplants in half lengthwise, puncturing skin in several places with a fork. Place, cut side down, on a lightly greased baking sheet. Bake until flesh is tender and skin is shriveled and blistered, about 25 to 35 minutes.

Remove from heat and cool. Remove skin from eggplants and discard. Drain pulp in a colander, pressing out as much of the liquid as possible. In a food processor, combine eggplant flesh, garlic, tahini, lemon juice, cumin, olive oil, black pepper and cayenne pepper until smooth. Taste, and adjust seasonings, adding more lemon juice if desired.

Place in a serving bowl and surround with cut-up raw vegetables.

Chutney Dip

Makes about 2 cups • Each 2 tablespoon serving: 5 grams protein • 9 grams carbohydrate

¾ cup sliced raw almonds

1 pound cream cheese, softened
at room temperature

1 cup Apricot and Raisin
Chutney (see recipe, page 287),
or store-bought chutney
(no sugar added)

2 teaspoons curry powder

½ teaspoon dried mustard

Put almonds in an ungreased medium skillet over medium-high heat. Stir nuts or shake pan almost constantly, until almonds are evenly browned and toasted. Remove from pan immediately and set aside.

In a food processor, blend cream cheese with ½ cup chutney, curry powder and mustard until smooth. Spoon into a bowl lined with plastic wrap. Fold plastic wrap over dip and seal. Refrigerate at least 2 hours.

Invert bowl onto serving platter and remove plastic wrap. Pour remaining chutney over top and sides of cheese spread. Sprinkle with toasted almonds and serve with cut-up raw vegetables.

Cream Cheese Pesto Dip

Makes about 1½ cups • Each 2 tablespoon serving: 5 grams protein • 2 grams carbohydrate

½ cup Basil Pesto (see recipe,
page 294) or store-bought

8 ounces cream cheese, softened
at room temperature

3 whole basil leaves, for garnish

In a small bowl, using a fork, combine pesto and cream cheese, blending until smooth; or blend in a food processor until smooth. Taste, and adjust seasonings.

To serve, mound dip in a small bowl and garnish with whole basil leaves. Serve with cut-up raw vegetables.

Famous Hot Artichoke Cheese Dip

Makes 8 servings • Each serving: 7 grams protein • 5 grams carbohydrate

13 ¾ ounces canned artichoke hearts in water, drained and rinsed

8 ounces cream cheese, diced into small cubes

⅓ cup mayonnaise (made from pure-pressed oil)

⅔ cup grated Parmesan cheese

2 tablespoons slivered fresh basil, or 1 teaspoon dried basil

1 teaspoon grated lemon zest

freshly ground black pepper, to taste

dash cayenne pepper

Preheat oven to 425°. Coarsely chop drained artichoke hearts. Mix with cream cheese, mayonnaise, Parmesan cheese, basil, lemon zest, black pepper and cayenne pepper. Transfer to a lightly oiled ovenproof casserole or 9-inch pie pan and bake about 20 minutes, until hot and bubbly. Serve with cut-up raw vegetables.

Garlic Herb Dip
with Toasted Walnuts

Makes about 1¼ cups • Each ¼ cup serving: 5 grams protein • 3 grams carbohydrate

½ cup chopped raw walnuts

8 ounces cream cheese, softened
  at room temperature

3 tablespoons fresh lemon juice

1 minced garlic clove

1 tablespoon finely chopped
  fresh parsley

1 teaspoon mixed dried Italian
  herbs (basil, oregano, thyme)

freshly ground black pepper,
  to taste

2 tablespoons all-dairy heavy
  cream

Put walnuts in an ungreased medium skillet, over medium-high heat. Stir nuts or shake pan almost constantly, until walnuts are evenly browned and toasted. Remove from pan immediately and set aside.

In a food processor, purée cream cheese with lemon juice, garlic, parsley, herbs, black pepper and cream until smooth. Put into a bowl, cover and refrigerate 2 hours.

To serve, sprinkle toasted walnuts on top. Surround dip with cut-up raw vegetables.

Gorgonzola Dip

Makes about 1³/₄ cups • Each ¼ cup serving: 6 grams protein • 1 gram carbohydrate
1 small apple: 15 grams carbohydrate • 1 small pear: 17 grams carbohydrate

4 ounces Gorgonzola or *any
  other blue-veined cheese*

*3 ounces cream cheese, softened
  at room temperature*

½ cup whole sour cream

¼ cup all-dairy heavy cream

1 tablespoon fresh lime juice

*2 tablespoons slivered fresh basil,
  or 1 teaspoon dried basil*

*freshly ground black pepper,
  to taste*

In a food processor purée all ingredients until smooth, or in a medium bowl, using a fork, mash Gorgonzola cheese with cream cheese. Add sour cream and heavy cream and blend until smooth. Gently mix in lime juice, basil and black pepper. Taste, and adjust seasonings. Transfer to a serving bowl, and surround with apple and pear slices and cut-up raw vegetables.

Guacamole

Makes about 2 cups • Each ¼ cup serving: 2 grams protein • 6 grams carbohydrate

3 ripe avocados

3 tablespoons minced red onion

1 minced garlic clove

2 tablespoons fresh lemon or lime
  juice

1 tablespoon chopped fresh
  cilantro

1 to 2 tablespoons salsa
  (see Salsas, starting on page
  296), or store-bought, or
  a few drops hot-pepper sauce

freshly ground black pepper,
  to taste

Cut avocados in half. Remove pits and scoop flesh into a medium bowl. Mash with a fork. Add remaining ingredients and mix well. Taste, and adjust seasonings.

Insert 1 avocado pit into mixture to prevent pulp from turning brown. Store covered in refrigerator. To serve, remove pit, mound in a small serving bowl and surround with cut-up raw vegetables.

Hummus

Makes about 2½ cups • Each ¼ cup serving: 7 grams protein • 16 grams carbohydrate

2 cans (30 ounces) garbanzo
  beans, drained and rinsed

2 minced garlic cloves

4 to 6 tablespoons fresh lemon
  juice, to taste

½ cup sesame tahini

¼ cup pure-pressed extra virgin
  olive oil

¼ to ½ cup water, as needed
  to thin

½ teaspoon ground cumin

cayenne pepper, to taste

paprika

In a food processor, combine drained beans with garlic, lemon juice, sesame tahini, olive oil, water, cumin and cayenne pepper until well blended. Taste, and adjust seasonings, adding more lemon juice if desired.

To serve, mound dip in a medium serving bowl. Sprinkle with paprika and surround with cut-up raw vegetables.

Ricotta Spinach Dip

Makes about 2½ cups • Each ¼ cup serving: 4 grams protein • 2 grams carbohydrate

1 bunch spinach equal to about
   1 cup cooked spinach, well
   drained and chopped; or
   8 ounces packaged frozen
   spinach, thawed, drained and
   chopped

1 cup whole ricotta cheese

½ cup whole sour cream

¼ cup chopped scallions

¼ cup chopped fresh parsley

1 teaspoon grated lemon zest

2 teaspoons fresh lemon juice

1 tablespoon minced fresh dill,
   or 1 teaspoon dried dill

freshly ground black pepper,
   to taste

dash cayenne pepper

In a food processor, purée all ingredients until creamy. Taste, and adjust seasonings. Refrigerate at least 1 hour before serving. Mound dip in small bowl and serve with cut-up raw vegetables.

Spreads

Chèvre (Goat Cheese) Spread

Makes about 2 cups • Each ¼ cup serving: 4 grams protein • 7 grams carbohydrate

1 cup sun-dried tomatoes in olive oil

½ cup chèvre (goat cheese)

1 cup coarsely chopped green olives

3 minced garlic cloves

2 tablespoons chopped fresh parsley

1 teaspoon grated lemon zest

freshly ground black pepper, to taste

In a blender or food processor, combine all ingredients, including oil from tomatoes, until smooth. Taste, and adjust seasonings. Mound dip in a small bowl and surround with cut-up raw vegetables.

Chèvre (Goat Cheese) with Pistachio Nuts

Makes about 1 cup • Each ¼ cup serving: 10 grams protein • 5 grams carbohydrate
1 small apple: 15 grams carbohydrate • 1 small pear: 17 grams carbohydrate

3 ounces chèvre (goat cheese)

3 ounces cream cheese, softened at room temperature

1 tablespoon all-dairy heavy cream

⅓ cup finely chopped dry-roasted pistachio nuts

dash cayenne pepper

¼ cup chopped dry-roasted pistachio nuts, for garnish

In a medium bowl, using a fork, blend chèvre (goat cheese), cream cheese, cream, chopped pistachio nuts and cayenne pepper. Transfer to a serving bowl and top with reserved pistachio nuts.

Spread on apple and pear slices or celery sticks.

Feta Cheese Spread
with Cucumber Rounds

Makes 6 servings • Each serving: 7 grams protein • 2 grams carbohydrate

½ pound crumbled feta cheese

1 tablespoon fresh lemon juice

1½ tablespoons pure-pressed extra virgin olive oil

6 finely chopped Kalamata olives

1 tablespoon finely chopped fresh parsley

1 tablespoon finely chopped red onion

2 tablespoons chopped dry-roasted pistachio nuts

freshly ground black pepper, to taste

1 hothouse English cucumber

extra whole dry-roasted pistachio nuts, for garnish

In a medium bowl, using a fork or your fingers, crumble feta cheese. Add lemon juice and olive oil and mix well. Add olives, parsley, red onion, chopped pistachio nuts and black pepper. Mix until well blended. Taste, and adjust seasonings.

Cut an unpeeled hothouse English cucumber into 1½-inch rounds. Using a melon-baller or small spoon, scoop out center flesh and seeds from one end of the round, leaving the other end intact. The rounds will now sit on a plate with a scooped-out cavity ready for filling. Spoon a tablespoon of feta filling into cavity. Garnish with a whole pistachio nut.

Pecan Baked Brie

Makes 8 servings • Each serving: 3 grams protein • trace carbohydrate
1 small apple: 15 grams carbohydrate • 1 small pear: 17 grams carbohydrate

8-ounce wheel of Brie cheese

1 tablespoon softened unsalted
*   butter*

¼ cup whole raw pecans

Preheat oven to 350°. Place Brie wheel in a lightly greased 8-inch glass pie pan or similar ovenproof dish. Spread butter over cheese, thoroughly covering white rind. Arrange whole pecans on top. Bake 10 to 12 minutes or until cheese begins to melt. Serve with apple and pear slices.

Quick Mushroom Paté Spread

Makes about 2 cups • Each ¼ cup serving: 2 grams protein • 3 grams carbohydrate

1 cup chopped raw walnuts

3 tablespoons unsalted butter

1 small finely chopped onion

1 minced clove garlic

½ pound chopped brown or white mushrooms

1 tablespoon low-sodium tamari soy sauce

freshly ground black pepper, to taste

1 tablespoon minced fresh parsley

Put walnuts in an ungreased medium skillet over medium-high heat. Stir nuts or shake pan almost constantly until walnuts are evenly browned and toasted. Remove from pan immediately and set aside to cool.

In a large nonstick saucepan, melt butter over medium-high heat. When butter is hot and bubbly, add onion and sauté until softened, about 5 minutes. Add mushrooms and sauté until softened and tender, about 5 minutes. Drain excess liquid from pan.

Transfer to a food processor. Add walnuts, soy sauce and black pepper. Purée until smooth. Taste, and adjust seasonings. Transfer to a serving bowl, sprinkle with parsley and surround with cut-up raw vegetables.

Sun-Dried Tomato Pesto

Makes about 1 cup • Each ¼ cup serving: 9 grams protein • 14 grams carbohydrate

1 cup sun-dried tomatoes in
  olive oil

2 tablespoons slivered fresh basil,
  or 1 teaspoon dried basil

¼ cup grated Parmesan cheese

1 minced garlic clove

⅛ teaspoon red-pepper flakes

In a blender or food processor, blend tomatoes with oil from jar, basil, Parmesan cheese, garlic and red-pepper flakes until smooth. Taste, and adjust seasonings.

Transfer to a serving bowl and serve at room temperature with cut-up raw vegetables.

Tangy Tofu and Peanut-Butter Stuffed Celery

Makes 6 servings • Each serving: 6 grams protein • 3 grams carbohydrate

1 tablespoon raw sesame seeds, for garnish

½ pound firm tofu, drained, pressed and crumbled (for directions, see "All You Need to Know About Tofu," page 10)

3 tablespoons organic peanut butter, creamy or crunchy (no honey or sugar added)

1 tablespoon sesame tahini

2 teaspoons low-sodium tamari soy sauce

1 tablespoon fresh lime juice

dash cayenne pepper

6 celery stalks, cut into 2-inch pieces

Put sesame seeds in an ungreased skillet over medium-high heat. Stir seeds or shake pan almost constantly until seeds are evenly browned and toasted and begin to pop. Remove from pan immediately and set aside.

In a food processor, combine tofu, peanut butter, sesame tahini, soy sauce, lime juice and cayenne pepper until creamy. Spoon into celery cavities and top with toasted sesame seeds.

Whole Roasted Garlic

Makes 6 servings • Each serving: trace protein • trace carbohydrate
Check packaging for nutritional analysis of crackers or bread.

3 whole large garlic bulbs

2 tablespoons pure-pressed extra
  virgin olive oil

freshly ground black pepper,
  to taste

Preheat oven to 425°. Peel off any loose outer layers of skin from whole garlic bulbs, leaving cloves intact and unpeeled. Slice off the top ½ inch of the bulbs and discard or reserve for another use.

Drizzle bulbs with olive oil and sprinkle with black pepper. Arrange on a lightly greased baking sheet and bake until cloves are browned and bursting out of their skins, about 20 minutes. Cool slightly. Squeeze pulp out of skins and spread on low-carbohydrate, whole-grain crackers or bread.

Soups

Bean and Grain Soups

Homemade Stock

Vegetable Soups

Bean and Grain Soups

To eat a balanced diet of all the essential nutrient groups, you must combine recipes. For example, if you prepare a soup that does not contain adequate protein, or contains too many carbohydrates, eat the soup as a side dish and prepare another protein dish to eat as a main course.

African Quinoa Soup with Vegetables

Makes 6 servings • Each serving: 11 grams protein • 24 grams carbohydrate

2 tablespoons unsalted butter

1 medium chopped onion

2 minced garlic cloves

1 small minced fresh jalapeño pepper; or 1 to 2 tablespoons canned diced green chilies, to taste [wear rubber gloves to prepare fresh jalapeño pepper]

1 diced red bell pepper

2 diced celery stalks with leaves

2 medium diced zucchini

1 medium diced sweet potato

1 teaspoon ground cumin

1 teaspoon dried oregano

6 cups vegetable stock (see recipe, page 100), or low-sodium canned

½ cup quinoa, rinsed and drained

freshly ground black pepper, to taste

dash cayenne pepper

½ cup chunky organic peanut butter (no honey or sugar added)

In a large heavy-bottomed soup pot, melt butter over medium-high heat. When butter is hot and bubbly, add onion, garlic, jalapeño pepper, bell pepper, celery, zucchini, sweet potato, cumin and oregano. Sauté 10 to 15 minutes, or until vegetables are softened.

Add stock, quinoa, black pepper and cayenne pepper. Bring to a boil, reduce heat and cover. Simmer until quinoa is cooked and vegetables are tender, about 10 to 15 minutes. Add peanut butter, using a wooden spoon to blend in completely, and simmer another 10 minutes. Taste, and adjust seasonings.

Black Bean Soup

Makes 6 servings • Each serving: 7 grams protein • 20 grams carbohydrate

2 cups dried black beans, picked over, rinsed and soaked overnight

2 tablespoons pure-pressed extra virgin olive oil

1 medium chopped red onion

3 minced garlic cloves

1 diced green or red bell pepper

½ cup chopped celery

½ cup diced carrots

1 teaspoon ground cumin

1 teaspoon chili powder

1 teaspoon dried oregano

2 bay leaves

14 ½ ounces canned tomatoes, chopped and peeled, with juice

freshly ground black pepper, to taste

3 tablespoons finely chopped fresh cilantro

dash hot-pepper sauce (optional)

1 to 2 tablespoons fresh lime juice, to taste

½ cup whole sour cream

Soak beans overnight by covering tops of beans with at least 4 inches of water. Drain and rinse well. Place beans in a large heavy-bottomed soup pot and cover with about 10 cups of fresh water. Bring to a boil. Reduce heat to medium and cook, uncovered, until tender, about 45 minutes to one hour, skimming off any foam that may collect on the surface.

In a large nonstick skillet, heat oil over medium-high heat. When oil is hot, add red onion, garlic, bell pepper, celery, carrots, cumin and chili powder, and sauté until softened, about 8 minutes. Add oregano, bay leaves, tomatoes and their juice. Stir well.

Add sautéed vegetable mixture to cooked beans and mix well. Cook over low heat 30 minutes, stirring occasionally, until beans are soft. Add more water if necessary. Remove bay leaves. Season to taste with black pepper. Stir in chopped cilantro, hot-pepper sauce and lime juice. Taste, and adjust seasonings. Blend until smooth in a blender or food processor, if desired. Serve with a spoonful of sour cream.

Moroccan Curried Lentil Soup

Makes 8 servings • Each serving: 10 grams protein • 18 grams carbohydrate

3 tablespoons unsalted butter

1 large diced onion

2 minced garlic cloves

1 diced green or red bell pepper

2 diced celery stalks with leaves

2 diced carrots

2 zucchini, quartered lengthwise, then diced into ½-inch cubes

1 teaspoon ground cumin

1 teaspoon ground curry powder

2 cups lentils, picked over and rinsed

8 cups vegetable stock (see recipe, page 100), or low-sodium canned

1 bay leaf

1 tablespoon peeled and finely minced fresh ginger

1 cup diced tomatoes

2 tablespoons finely chopped fresh cilantro

freshly ground black pepper, to taste

1 tablespoon fresh lemon juice

In a large heavy-bottomed soup pot, melt butter over medium-high heat. When butter is hot and bubbly, add onion, garlic and bell pepper and cook until softened, about 5 minutes. Add celery, carrots, zucchini, cumin and curry powder and sauté 5 minutes. Add lentils, stock and bay leaf. Bring to a boil, reduce heat, and simmer over low heat, covered, 30 to 45 minutes, or until lentils are tender. Add ginger, tomatoes, cilantro and black pepper. Simmer another 15 minutes to blend flavors. Add lemon juice. Taste, and adjust seasonings.

Mushroom Barley Soup

Makes 6 servings • Each serving: 8 grams protein • 17 grams carbohydrate

3 tablespoons unsalted butter

1 medium chopped onion

2 minced garlic cloves

2 diced celery stalks with leaves

2 diced carrots

2 teaspoons dried oregano

1 teaspoon dried thyme

2 bay leaves

½ cup pearl barley, rinsed and drained

6 cups vegetable stock (see recipe, page 100), or low-sodium canned

2 tablespoons unsalted butter

¾ pound thinly sliced brown or white mushrooms

1 cup fresh green peas or frozen and thawed

freshly ground black pepper, to taste

2 tablespoons finely chopped fresh parsley, for garnish

In a large heavy-bottomed soup pot, melt butter over medium-high heat. When butter is hot and bubbly, add onion and garlic and cook until softened, about 5 minutes. Add celery, carrots, oregano, thyme, bay leaves and barley, and stir until well blended.

Add stock and bring to a boil. Reduce heat to low. Cover and simmer until barley is tender, about 45 minutes.

In a large saucepan, melt butter over medium-high heat. When butter is hot and bubbly, add sliced mushrooms and sauté until softened and their liquid has been released, about 5 minutes. Add mushrooms to soup pot along with peas and black pepper. Simmer over low heat 5 minutes or until peas are tender. Taste, and adjust seasonings. Serve garnished with finely chopped parsley.

Vegetable Split-Pea Soup

Makes 6 servings • Each serving: 8 grams protein • 9 grams carbohydrate

*1 cup split peas, picked over
and rinsed*

*6 cups vegetable stock (see recipe,
page 100), or low-sodium
canned, or water*

*2 tablespoons pure-pressed extra
virgin olive oil*

1 medium finely chopped onion

2 minced garlic cloves

2 diced celery stalks with leaves

2 diced carrots

1 teaspoon ground cumin

1 teaspoon dried oregano

2 bay leaves

*2 tablespoons minced fresh
parsley*

*freshly ground black pepper,
to taste*

dash red-pepper flakes

*1 to 2 tablespoons fresh lemon
juice, to taste*

In a large heavy-bottomed soup pot, bring split peas and stock or water to a boil over high heat. Reduce heat to low, cover and simmer 30 minutes, skimming off any foam that may collect on the surface.

In a large nonstick skillet, heat oil over medium-high heat. When oil is hot, add onion, garlic, celery, carrots, cumin, oregano, bay leaves, parsley, black pepper and red-pepper flakes. Cook until vegetables have softened, about 8 minutes, stirring occasionally.

Add sautéed vegetables to soup pot and simmer, uncovered, 1 hour, or until peas are soft, stirring occasionally. Remove bay leaves. In a blender or food processor, purée soup in batches until smooth. Add lemon juice. Taste, and adjust seasonings.

Homemade Stock

Vegetable Stock

After straining, makes about 3 quarts.
Each 1 cup serving: 4 grams protein • 6 grams carbohydrate

2 large quartered onions

*2 large well-washed coarsely
  chopped leeks*

4 carrots, cut into 2-inch pieces

*4 celery stalks with leaves, cut
  into 2-inch pieces*

*2 medium zucchini, cut into
  1-inch rounds*

*2 parsnips, cut into 2-inch
  chunks*

4 to 5 fresh thyme sprigs, or
  2 teaspoons dried thyme leaves

6 to 12 whole black peppercorns

1 bunch fresh parsley

4 quarts water

**plus any optional vegetables
on hand, such as:**

*½ pound quartered brown or
  white mushrooms*

1 chopped bell pepper

*any shredded greens, such as
  spinach* or *Swiss chard*

In a large heavy-bottomed stock pot, bring all ingredients to a boil over high heat. Reduce heat to low and simmer, uncovered, 45 minutes. Using a fine-meshed sieve, strain stock and discard vegetables. Refrigerate or freeze for future use.

Vegetable Soups

Anytime Soup is a "prescription" soup to eat during the initial phase of the Healing Program as described in *The Schwarzbein Principle*. If you are hungry *between meals*, eat Anytime Soup as a snack.

Anytime Soup

Makes 6 servings • Each serving: 4 grams protein • 10 grams carbohydrate

½ small head shredded green cabbage

1 minced garlic clove

2 chopped celery stalks with leaves

2 pounds medium diced fresh tomatoes

3 chopped carrots

2 tablespoons chopped fresh parsley

½ teaspoon dried thyme

½ teaspoon dried basil

freshly ground black pepper, to taste

4 cups vegetable stock (see recipe, page 100), or low-sodium canned

1 to 2 tablespoons fresh lemon juice, or 1 to 2 tablespoons cider vinegar, to taste

In a large heavy-bottomed soup pot, bring all ingredients, *except* lemon juice or vinegar to a boil. Lower heat and simmer 20 to 30 minutes, until vegetables are softened. Add lemon juice or vinegar.

Broccoli Potato Cheese Soup

Makes 6 servings • Each serving: 8 grams protein • 12 grams carbohydrate

4 tablespoons unsalted butter

1 well-washed diced leek

1 minced garlic clove

1 diced carrot

3 diced medium red potatoes
(peeled, if desired)

4 cups vegetable stock (see recipe,
page 100), or low-sodium
canned

1 bay leaf

½ teaspoon celery seed

2 sprigs fresh thyme, or
1 teaspoon dried thyme

¼ cup slivered fresh basil, or
2 teaspoons dried basil

1 bunch broccoli, cut into
bite-size florets, with stalks
peeled and chopped

1 cup all-dairy heavy cream

freshly ground black pepper,
to taste

dash cayenne pepper

1 cup grated Monterey Jack
cheese

whole basil leaves, for garnish

In a large heavy-bottomed soup pot, melt butter over medium-high heat. When butter is hot and bubbly, add leeks, garlic and carrots and cook until softened, about 5 minutes. Add potatoes, stir well and cook 2 minutes.

Add stock, bay leaf, celery seed, thyme and basil. Bring to a boil. Reduce heat to low and cook until potatoes are barely tender, about 15 minutes. Add broccoli and cook about another 10 minutes, until tender.

In a blender or food processor, purée soup in batches until vegetables are well blended. Pour soup back into pot and stir in cream. Season to taste with black pepper and cayenne pepper. Cook over low heat until heated through. *Do not boil.* Stir in cheese just before serving. Taste, and adjust seasonings. Garnish with fresh basil leaves.

Cauliflower Potato Soup

Makes 4 servings • Each serving: 7 grams protein • 18 grams carbohydrate

2 tablespoons unsalted butter

1 medium chopped onion

1 minced garlic clove

4 medium diced red potatoes
(peeled, if desired)

½ cup diced celery

4 cups vegetable stock (see recipe,
page 100), or low-sodium
canned

1 medium head cauliflower,
cut into florets

2 tablespoons slivered fresh basil,
or 2 teaspoons dried basil

1 tablespoon minced fresh parsley

½ cup fresh green peas or frozen
and thawed

freshly ground black pepper,
to taste

½ cup all-dairy heavy cream

In a large heavy-bottomed soup pot, melt butter over medium-high
heat. When butter is hot and bubbly, add onion and garlic and sauté
until softened, about 5 minutes. Add potatoes and celery and stir,
cooking about 2 minutes. Add stock and bring to a boil. Reduce heat
to low. Cover and simmer until potatoes are almost tender, about 10
minutes. Add cauliflower and cook 7 minutes, or until tender.

Add basil, parsley, peas, black pepper and cream. Simmer over low
heat until heated through. *Do not boil.* Taste, and adjust seasonings.
Serve chunky-style, or purée in a blender or food processor until
creamy.

Chinese Bean Curd Soup

Makes 6 servings • Each serving: 12 grams protein • 5 grams carbohydrate

2 tablespoons pure-pressed
  peanut oil

2 minced garlic cloves

2 teaspoons peeled and finely
  minced fresh ginger

¼ pound Chinese snow peas or
  sugar snap peas, ends trimmed

1 cup thinly sliced brown or
  white mushrooms

6 cups vegetable stock (see recipe,
  page 100), or low-sodium
  canned

2 to 3 tablespoons low-sodium
  tamari soy sauce, to taste

2 beaten eggs

½ pound firm tofu, drained,
  pressed and cut into ½-inch
  cubes (for directions, see
  "All You Need to Know About
  Tofu," page 10)

freshly ground black pepper,
  to taste

2 tablespoons finely chopped
  scallions, for garnish

In a large heavy-bottomed soup pot, heat oil over medium-high heat. When oil is hot, add garlic, ginger, snow peas and mushrooms, and stir-fry until snow peas turn bright green, about 2 minutes. Add vegetable stock and soy sauce. Bring to a boil.

Using chopsticks or a fork, stir quickly while pouring in beaten eggs in a steady stream. Add cubed tofu. Remove from heat. Season to taste with black pepper. Sprinkle with chopped scallions.

Cream of Mushroom Soup

Makes 4 servings • Each serving: 5 grams protein • 6 grams carbohydrate

2 tablespoons unsalted butter

1 cup minced onion

1 minced garlic clove

1 pound thinly sliced brown or white mushrooms

1 tablespoon flour

4 cups vegetable stock (see recipe, page 100), or low-sodium canned

1 tablespoon finely chopped fresh parsley

1 bay leaf

¼ teaspoon nutmeg, or ½ teaspoon dried thyme

dash cayenne pepper

1 cup all-dairy heavy cream

4 sprigs fresh parsley, for garnish

In a large heavy-bottomed soup pot, melt butter over medium-high heat. When butter is hot and bubbly, add onion and garlic and sauté until softened, about 5 minutes. Add mushrooms and cook until they release their liquid and soften, about 5 minutes.

Sprinkle flour over onion and mushroom mixture and cook over low heat, stirring, 3 to 4 minutes. Gradually add stock, parsley, bay leaf, nutmeg or thyme and cayenne pepper. Bring to a boil, stirring constantly. Reduce heat and simmer gently 20 minutes, stirring occasionally. Stir in cream. Simmer until heated through. *Do not boil.*

Taste, and adjust seasonings. Garnish bowls with a sprig of fresh parsley.

Creamy Artichoke Chowder

Makes 4 servings • Each serving: 7 grams protein • 15 grams carbohydrate

2 tablespoons pure-pressed extra
  virgin olive oil

½ cup chopped onion

2 minced garlic cloves

2 cups sliced brown or white
  mushrooms

13¾ ounces canned artichoke
  hearts in water, drained and
  chopped

1 teaspoon dried thyme

1 tablespoon slivered fresh basil,
  or 1 teaspoon dried basil

3 cups vegetable stock (see recipe,
  page 100), or low-sodium
  canned

1 cup fresh green peas or frozen
  and thawed

1 cup all-dairy heavy cream

freshly ground black pepper,
  to taste

In a large heavy-bottomed soup pot, heat oil over medium-high heat. When oil is hot, add onion and garlic and sauté until softened, about 5 minutes. Add mushrooms, artichokes, thyme and basil and sauté 5 minutes.

Add vegetable stock. Bring to a boil. Reduce heat to low and add peas, cream and black pepper. Cook until heated through and peas are tender. *Do not boil.* Taste, and adjust seasonings.

Creamy Broccoli Soup

Makes 6 servings • Each serving: 4 grams protein • 6 grams carbohydrate

3 tablespoons unsalted butter

1 medium finely chopped onion

1 chopped celery stalk with
    leaves

1 diced carrot

5 cups vegetable stock (see recipe,
    page 100), or low-sodium
    canned

1 bunch broccoli cut into florets,
    with stalks, peeled and chopped

2 tablespoons slivered fresh basil,
    or 2 teaspoons dried basil

1 teaspoon dried thyme

freshly ground black pepper,
    to taste

1 cup all-dairy heavy cream

In a large heavy-bottomed soup pot, melt butter over medium-high heat. When butter is hot and bubbly, add onion and sauté until softened, about 5 minutes. Add celery and carrot and sauté 5 minutes, stirring occasionally.

Add stock, broccoli, basil, thyme and black pepper. Bring to a boil. Cover, reduce heat to low and simmer until vegetables are tender, about 7 minutes. Remove from heat.

Add cream and mix well. In a blender or food processor, purée soup in batches until smooth and creamy. Taste, and adjust seasonings. Reheat over low heat. *Do not boil.*

Creamy Roasted Eggplant Soup

Makes 4 servings • Each serving: 6 grams protein • 17 grams carbohydrate

2 medium eggplants

1 red bell pepper or ¼ cup store-bought roasted red bell pepper

2 tablespoons unsalted butter

1 medium diced onion

1 minced garlic clove

4 cups vegetable stock (see recipe, page 100), or low-sodium canned

3 tablespoons Basil or Cilantro Pesto (see recipes, page 294) or store-bought

1 cup all-dairy heavy cream

freshly ground black pepper, to taste

dash cayenne pepper

whole fresh cilantro sprigs, for garnish

Preheat oven to 425°. Cut eggplant in half lengthwise, puncturing skin in several places with a fork. Place cut-side down, on a lightly greased baking sheet. Bake until flesh is tender and skin is shriveled and blistered, about 25 to 35 minutes. Remove from heat and cool. Remove skin from eggplant and discard. Drain pulp in a colander, pressing out as much liquid as possible. Chop eggplant pulp coarsely. Set aside.

If using a fresh red bell pepper, roast pepper directly over a gas flame or under preheated broiler on a broiler rack. Using tongs, turn pepper frequently, until blistered and blackened on all sides. Place pepper in a bowl with a plate on top. Let steam for 15 minutes to loosen skin. Peel off all charred skin. Discard skin and seeds. Dice flesh and set aside.

In a large heavy-bottomed soup pot, melt butter over medium-high heat. When butter is hot and bubbly, add onion and garlic and sauté until softened, about 5 minutes. Add diced, roasted red pepper and chopped eggplant. Add vegetable stock and bring to a boil. Reduce heat to low and simmer 20 minutes.

In a blender or food processor, purée soup in batches until smooth. Return purée to soup pot and stir in Basil or Cilantro Pesto and cream. Season to taste with black pepper and cayenne pepper. Taste, and adjust seasonings. Reheat over low heat. *Do not boil.* Garnish with whole cilantro sprigs.

Creamy Spinach Soup

Makes 4 servings • Each serving: 6 grams protein • 8 grams carbohydrate

4 bunches spinach equal to about
 4 cups cooked spinach, well
 drained and chopped; or
 32 ounces packaged frozen
 spinach, thawed, drained
 and chopped

4 tablespoons unsalted butter

1 medium diced onion

1 minced garlic clove

1 tablespoon flour

1 teaspoon Dijon mustard

4 cups vegetable stock (see recipe,
 page 100), or low-sodium
 canned

1½ cups all-dairy heavy cream

¼ cup slivered fresh basil, or
 2 teaspoons dried basil

freshly ground black pepper,
 to taste

dash cayenne pepper

whole basil leaves, for garnish

Wash spinach well, removing stems. With water still clinging to leaves, place in a medium saucepan with a tight-fitting lid. Turn heat to medium-high and steam until leaves are wilted, about 2 to 3 minutes. Drain in a colander, pressing out all liquid with the back of a wooden spoon. Chop fine and set aside.

In a heavy-bottomed soup pot, melt butter over medium-high heat. When butter is hot and bubbly, add onion and garlic and sauté until softened, about 5 minutes.

Reduce heat to low, sprinkle in flour and cook 3 to 4 minutes, stirring. *Do not brown.* Stir in mustard and stock. Blend well. Bring to a boil, reduce heat to low and cook until slightly thickened and smooth, about 15 minutes. Add cream, chopped spinach, basil, black pepper and cayenne pepper. Mix well.

In a blender or food processor, purée soup in batches until smooth and creamy. Return puréed soup to soup pot and cook over low heat until heated through. *Do not boil.* Taste, and adjust seasonings. Serve garnished with whole basil leaves.

Creamy Tomato Soup

Makes 4 servings • Each serving: 7 grams protein • 21 grams carbohydrate

3 pounds fresh tomatoes, peeled, seeded and finely chopped*; or 28 ounces canned plum tomatoes, with juice

1 tablespoon pure-pressed extra virgin olive oil

1 tablespoon unsalted butter

1 medium diced onion

2 minced garlic cloves

1 diced carrot

1 diced celery stalk with leaves

½ cup sun-dried tomatoes in olive oil, drained and chopped

¼ cup finely chopped fresh parsley

⅓ cup slivered fresh basil, or 2 teaspoons dried basil

1 bay leaf

3 cups vegetable stock (see recipe, page 100), or low-sodium canned

freshly ground black pepper, to taste

1 cup all-dairy heavy cream

In a large heavy-bottomed soup pot, heat oil and butter over medium-high heat. When hot, add onion, garlic, carrots and celery. Sauté until vegetables are softened, about 5 minutes. Add tomatoes and their juice, sun-dried tomatoes, parsley, basil, bay leaf, stock and black pepper. Slowly bring to a boil. Reduce heat to low, partially cover, and simmer 30 minutes, stirring occasionally.

Remove bay leaf. In a blender or food processor, purée soup in batches, until smooth. Return soup to pot and stir in cream. Taste, and adjust seasonings. Simmer until heated through, about 5 minutes. *Do not boil.*

---

* To peel and seed tomatoes: Plunge tomatoes into boiling water for about 20 seconds, then into cold water. Skins will slip off easily. Cut tomatoes in half and gently squeeze. Scoop out seeds with a small spoon or your fingers. Chop tomatoes.

Italian Mixed Vegetable Soup

Makes 6 servings • Each serving: 10 grams protein • 26 grams carbohydrate

2 tablespoons pure-pressed extra virgin olive oil

1 medium finely chopped onion

1 minced garlic clove

1 diced green or red bell pepper

1 chopped celery stalk with leaves

1 diced carrot

1 large diced red potato (peeled, if desired)

¼ pound green beans, ends trimmed, sliced diagonally into 1-inch pieces

1 medium diced zucchini

*28 ounces canned peeled plum tomatoes, chopped (*reserve liquid*)*

4 cups vegetable stock (see recipe, page 100), or *low-sodium canned*

2 bay leaves

1 teaspoon dried oregano

1 teaspoon dried basil

1 teaspoon dried marjoram

freshly ground black pepper, to taste

13¾ ounces canned pinto beans, drained and rinsed

2 tablespoons chopped fresh parsley

2 tablespoons grated Parmesan cheese, for topping

In a large heavy-bottomed soup pot, heat oil over medium-high heat. When oil is hot, add onion, garlic and bell pepper and sauté until softened, about 5 minutes. Add celery, carrot, potato and green beans. Cook, stirring occasionally, 5 minutes. Add zucchini, tomatoes and their liquid, stock, bay leaves, oregano, basil, marjoram and black pepper. Bring to a boil. Reduce heat to low and simmer, covered, until vegetables are tender, about 15 to 20 minutes. Add pinto beans and parsley and cook until heated through. Taste, and adjust seasonings.

Sprinkle with Parmesan cheese before serving.

Miso Soup

Makes 6 servings • Each serving: 13 grams protein • 8 grams carbohydrate

6 cups vegetable stock (see recipe, page 100), or low-sodium canned

½ cup miso

½ pound firm tofu, drained, pressed and cut into ½-inch cubes (for directions, see "All You Need to Know About Tofu," page 10)

¼ pound fresh spinach, washed, drained and shredded

8 thinly sliced brown or white mushrooms

¼ cup diced scallions

In a large soup pot, bring vegetable stock to a boil. Remove 1 cup of hot liquid to a small bowl. Using a fork, mix liquid with miso until smooth and lump-free. Return diluted miso to pot and mix well, reducing heat to low. Add tofu, shredded spinach and mushrooms, and cook until heated through, about 2 minutes. Ladle into bowls and sprinkle scallions on top.

Spicy Sweet Potato Soup

Makes 4 servings • Each serving: 5 grams protein • 24 grams carbohydrate

2 tablespoons unsalted butter

1 medium chopped onion

1 small diced fresh jalapeño pepper; or 1 to 2 tablespoons canned diced green chilies, to taste [wear rubber gloves to prepare fresh jalapeño pepper]

3 sweet potatoes, peeled and diced into 1-inch cubes

1 teaspoon ground cumin

freshly ground black pepper, to taste

3 cups vegetable stock (see recipe, page 100), or low-sodium canned

1 cup all-dairy heavy cream

2 tablespoons fresh lime juice

2 tablespoons minced fresh parsley or cilantro, for garnish

In a large heavy-bottomed soup pot, melt butter over medium-high heat. When butter is hot and bubbly, add onion and jalapeño pepper and sauté until softened, about 5 minutes. Add cubed sweet potatoes, cumin and black pepper and sauté 10 minutes. Add vegetable stock and bring to a boil. Reduce heat to low and simmer until potatoes are tender, about 15 minutes.

In a blender, purée soup in batches with cream until smooth and creamy. Add lime juice and reheat over low heat. *Do not boil.* Taste, and adjust seasonings. Ladle into bowls and sprinkle with minced parsley or cilantro.

Very French Onion Soup

Makes 6 servings • Each serving: 9 grams protein • 4 grams carbohydrate

3 tablespoons unsalted butter

4 large thinly sliced red onions

1 minced garlic clove

6 cups vegetable stock (see recipe, page 100), or low-sodium canned

½ teaspoon dried thyme

freshly ground black pepper, to taste

1 cup grated Gruyère cheese

¼ cup grated Parmesan cheese

In a heavy-bottomed soup pot, melt butter over medium-high heat. When butter is hot and bubbly, add onion and garlic and sauté over medium-low heat, stirring occasionally, until well softened, about 30 minutes.

Add vegetable stock, thyme and black pepper. Bring to a boil, reduce heat to low, and simmer, uncovered, 30 minutes. Taste, and adjust seasonings.

Preheat broiler. Divide soup into 6 ovenproof serving bowls. Top with Gruyère and Parmesan cheeses. Place on top rack of oven and broil until cheese is bubbly and melted.

Vichyssoise
(Cold Potato Soup)

Makes 4 servings • Each serving: 6 grams protein • 21 grams carbohydrate

3 tablespoons unsalted butter

2 large well-washed thinly sliced
  leeks

3 medium diced red potatoes
  (peeled, if desired)

4 cups vegetable stock (see recipe,
  page 100), or low-sodium
  canned

2 tablespoons slivered fresh basil,
  or 2 teaspoons dried basil

freshly ground black pepper,
  to taste

1 cup all-dairy heavy cream

2 tablespoons minced fresh
  chives, or finely chopped
  scallions

In a large heavy-bottomed soup pot, melt butter over medium-high heat. When butter is hot and bubbly, add leeks and sauté until softened, about 5 minutes.

Add potatoes and sauté until well-coated with butter, about 1 minute. Add stock and bring to a boil. Reduce heat to low. Cover and simmer until potatoes are tender, about 10 to 15 minutes. Add basil and black pepper.

In a blender or food processor, purée soup in batches until smooth and creamy. Chill soup. Add cream just before serving. Taste, and adjust seasonings. Sprinkle bowls with chopped chives or scallions.

This soup is also delicious served hot. To serve hot: Purée soup with cream. Return to pot to reheat. *Do not boil.*

Salads

Vegetable Salads

Vegetable Salads

Beet and Onion Salad

Makes 4 side-dish servings • Each serving: 2 grams protein • 11 grams carbohydrate

*1 pound fresh steamed, peeled
   and julienned beets*

1 medium thinly sliced red onion

*3 tablespoons slivered fresh basil,
   or 3 tablespoons minced fresh
   parsley*

Beet Vinaigrette

Combine beets, onion and fresh basil or parsley. Pour Beet Vinaigrette over salad and refrigerate 30 minutes before serving.

Beet Vinaigrette

1 tablespoon balsamic vinegar

1 tablespoon red wine vinegar

*3 tablespoons pure-pressed extra
   virgin olive oil*

*freshly ground black pepper,
   to taste*

In a small bowl, using a fork, whisk vinegars, oil and black pepper until smooth.

California Coleslaw

Makes 4 side-dish servings • Each serving: 2 grams protein • trace carbohydrate

1 ½ cups shredded green
   cabbage

1 ½ cups shredded red cabbage

1 coarsely grated carrot

3 celery stalks, sliced thin
   diagonally

½ thinly sliced red onion
   (optional)

¼ cup minced fresh parsley

California Coleslaw Dressing

In a large bowl, toss all ingredients with California Coleslaw Dressing. Refrigerate at least 1 hour before serving.

California Coleslaw Dressing

½ cup mayonnaise (made from
   pure-pressed oil)

¼ cup red wine vinegar

½ teaspoon celery seed

1 teaspoon Dijon mustard

2 tablespoons minced fresh
   parsley

freshly ground black pepper,
   to taste

In a blender or food processor, blend all ingredients until smooth; or place ingredients in a jar with a tight-fitting lid and shake vigorously until well blended. Taste, and adjust seasonings.

Caponata Salad

Makes 6 side-dish servings • Each serving: 4 grams protein • 4 grams carbohydrate

2 tablespoons raw pine nuts,
for garnish

¼ cup pure-pressed extra virgin
olive oil

1 medium eggplant, cut into
½-inch cubes (peeled, if desired)

2 tablespoons extra virgin olive oil

3 minced garlic cloves

1 medium chopped red onion

3 chopped celery stalks

1 chopped red bell pepper

one 14-ounce can plum tomatoes,
drained and chopped (reserve
liquid)

2 tablespoons drained and rinsed
capers

½ cup pitted and chopped green
olives

1 bay leaf

1 tablespoon chopped fresh
parsley

1 tablespoon balsamic vinegar

½ teaspoon dried oregano

½ teaspoon dried basil

freshly ground black pepper,
to taste

Put pine nuts in an ungreased skillet, over medium-high heat. Stir nuts or shake pan almost constantly, until pine nuts are evenly browned and toasted. Remove from pan immediately and set aside.

In a large nonstick skillet, heat ¼ cup oil over medium-high heat. When oil is hot, add eggplant and sauté until softened and lightly browned, about 10 minutes. Remove from skillet and set aside.

In the same skillet, heat remaining 2 tablespoons oil over medium-high heat. When oil is hot, add garlic, onion, celery and bell pepper, and sauté until softened, about 8 minutes. Add chopped tomatoes, cooked eggplant, capers, olives, bay leaf, parsley, vinegar, oregano, basil and black pepper. Simmer over low heat 20 to 30 minutes, stirring occasionally. Add reserved tomato liquid, if needed, to prevent sticking. Taste, and adjust seasonings.

Spoon into a serving bowl and garnish with toasted pine nuts. Serve at room temperature.

Carrot Salad

Makes 8 side-dish servings • Each serving: 1 gram protein • 1 gram carbohydrate

1 pound shredded carrots	*½ cup diced raw walnuts*
1 fennel bulb (stalk and core removed), cut into lengthwise thin strips	*½ cup chopped fresh parsley* *Carrot Salad Dressing*

Combine carrots, fennel, walnuts and parsley. Toss with Carrot Salad Dressing and marinate in refrigerator 1 hour before serving.

Carrot Salad Dressing

3 tablespoons fresh lime juice	*2 tablespoons pure-pressed extra virgin olive oil*
1 teaspoon ground cumin	
freshly ground black pepper, to taste	

In a small bowl, using a fork, whisk lime juice, cumin and black pepper. Slowly drizzle in olive oil, whisking until smooth. Taste, and adjust seasonings.

Classic Egg Salad

Makes 4 servings • Each serving: 16 grams protein • trace carbohydrate

8 hard-boiled eggs

1 tablespoon Dijon mustard

½ cup mayonnaise (made from pure-pressed oil)

1 tablespoon capers, rinsed and drained (optional)

1 tablespoon minced fresh parsley

½ teaspoon dried dill

freshly ground black pepper, to taste

dash cayenne pepper

To hard boil eggs, place eggs in a saucepan and cover with cold water. Bring to boil uncovered. Allow to boil for one minute, then cover, remove from heat, and let sit undisturbed for 10 minutes. Rinse eggs under cold water. Crack shells, peel and rinse eggs and chop fine.

In a medium bowl combine chopped egg with remaining ingredients. Taste, and adjust seasonings.

Classic Tomato and Mozzarella Salad

Makes 4 side-dish servings • Each serving: 9 grams protein • 6 grams carbohydrate

4 firm, large, very ripe tomatoes

½ pound sliced fresh Buffalo
  mozzarella cheese

¼ cup slivered fresh basil, or
  2 teaspoons dried basil

Classic Vinaigrette

Thinly slice tomatoes and arrange on plates, alternating with mozzarella slices. Sprinkle with fresh basil. Spoon Classic Vinaigrette over salad. Refrigerate 1 hour before serving.

Classic Vinaigrette

2 tablespoons red wine vinegar

3 tablespoons pure-pressed extra
  virgin olive oil

freshly ground black pepper,
  to taste

In a small bowl, using a fork, whisk all ingredients until well blended.

Cottage Cheese Salad with Chopped Vegetables

Makes 4 side-dish servings • Each serving: 15 grams protein • 3 grams carbohydrate

2 finely diced carrots

3 finely chopped scallions

1 finely chopped red bell pepper

3 finely chopped celery stalks

1 tablespoon minced fresh parsley

1 tablespoon minced fresh chives

2 cups whole cottage cheese

freshly ground black pepper,
  to taste

4 cups mixed salad greens

In a medium bowl, using a fork, mix all ingredients, except salad greens, with cottage cheese. Line 4 individual plates with mixed salad greens. Mound cottage cheese salad on top. Serve immediately.

Creamy Marinated Cucumbers

Makes 4 side-dish servings • Each serving: 3 grams protein • 2 grams carbohydrate

3 medium cucumbers, regular	*½ teaspoon salt*
or hothouse	*Creamy Cucumber Marinade*

If using regular waxed cucumbers, peel, cut in half lengthwise, remove seeds and slice into thin half-circles. If using unwaxed hothouse cucumbers, score flesh by running the tines of a fork down sides, making deep incisions. Slice into thin circles. Sprinkle cucumber slices with salt and toss well to coat. Let cucumbers drain about 30 minutes in a colander. Rinse well under cold water to remove salt and pat dry with paper towels. Toss with Creamy Cucumber Marinade and marinate 30 minutes before serving.

Creamy Cucumber Marinade

⅔ cup whole sour cream	*1 minced garlic clove*
2 teaspoons minced fresh mint	*2 tablespoons fresh lemon juice*
2 teaspoons minced fresh parsley	*freshly ground black pepper,*
2 teaspoons minced scallions	*to taste*

In a medium bowl, using a fork, whisk dressing ingredients. Toss with drained cucumbers. Taste, and adjust seasonings.

Curried Spinach Salad with Almond Dressing

Makes 4 side-dish servings • Each serving: 8 grams protein • 19 grams carbohydrate

1 diced carrot	*2 diced celery stalks*
1 diced green apple	*⅓ cup raisins*
6 cups washed and dried spinach leaves	*Curried Almond Dressing*

In a large bowl, combine carrot, apple, celery and raisins. Arrange spinach leaves on 4 individual salad plates. Mound carrot mixture on top of spinach. Serve Curried Almond Dressing on the side.

Curried Almond Dressing

½ cup coarsely chopped raw almonds	*1 tablespoon sesame tahini*
⅔ cup pure-pressed extra virgin olive oil	*1 minced garlic clove*
½ cup fresh lime juice	*¼ cup mayonnaise (made from pure-pressed oil)*
2 tablespoons fresh orange juice	*½ teaspoon curry powder*
2 teaspoons low-sodium tamari soy sauce	*freshly ground black pepper, to taste*

Put almonds in an ungreased skillet over medium-high heat. Stir or shake pan almost constantly, until almonds are evenly browned and toasted. Remove from pan immediately and set aside.

In a blender or food processor, combine all ingredients with ¼ cup toasted almonds and blend until smooth; or place ingredients in a jar with a tight-fitting lid and shake vigorously until well blended. Stir in remaining almonds. Taste, and adjust seasonings.

Garbanzo Bean Salad

Makes 4 side-dish servings • Each serving: 6 grams protein • 8 grams carbohydrate

13¾ ounces canned garbanzo
  beans, drained and rinsed
½ cup chopped red onion
1 cup diced celery stalks
1 cup diced carrot

½ cup minced fresh parsley
1 cup seeded and diced cucumber
1 cup diced red bell pepper
Garbanzo Vinaigrette

In a large bowl, toss all ingredients with Garbanzo Vinaigrette. Cover, and chill 1 hour before serving.

Garbanzo Vinaigrette

1 minced garlic clove
2 tablespoons fresh lemon juice
2 tablespoons balsamic vinegar
1 tablespoon Dijon mustard

4 tablespoons pure-pressed extra
  virgin olive oil
freshly ground black pepper,
  to taste

In a blender or food processor, combine all ingredients and blend until smooth; or place ingredients in a jar with a tight-fitting lid and shake vigorously until well blended. Taste, and adjust seasonings.

Greek Salad

Makes 4 side-dish servings • Each serving: 12 grams protein • 3 grams carbohydrate

1 head romaine lettuce, washed, dried and torn into bite-size pieces

2 tomatoes, cut into chunks

2 cups green beans, ends trimmed, sliced into 1-inch pieces and steamed until just tender, and cooled to room temperature

12 Kalamata or any style Greek olives

1 peeled and sliced cucumber

½ thinly sliced red onion

1 cup crumbled feta cheese

2 tablespoons minced fresh parsley, for garnish

Greek Dressing

Line a platter with washed and dried lettuce. Arrange remaining ingredients, except parsley, on top of lettuce. Toss lightly with Greek Dressing. Sprinkle with parsley.

Greek Dressing

2 tablespoons red wine vinegar

1 minced garlic clove

1 tablespoon fresh lemon juice

1 teaspoon Dijon mustard

1 teaspoon dried oregano

½ cup pure-pressed extra virgin olive oil

freshly ground black pepper, to taste

In a blender or food processor, combine all ingredients and blend until smooth; or place ingredients in a jar with a tight-fitting lid and shake vigorously until well blended. Taste, and adjust seasonings.

Green Bean, Feta Cheese and Kalamata Olive Salad

Makes 4 side-dish servings • Each serving: 9 grams protein • 2 grams carbohydrate

1 pound fresh green beans, ends
  trimmed, sliced diagonally into
  1-inch pieces and steamed
  until tender

½ thinly sliced red onion

⅔ cup pitted and diced Kalamata
  olives

⅔ cup crumbled feta cheese

¼ cup slivered fresh basil, or
  2 teaspoons dried basil

Dijon Garlic Marinade

Combine all ingredients and mix with Dijon Garlic Marinade.

Dijon Garlic Marinade

3 tablespoons balsamic vinegar

1 tablespoon Dijon mustard

2 minced garlic cloves

freshly ground black pepper,
  to taste

3 tablespoons pure-pressed extra
  virgin olive oil

In a small bowl, using a fork, combine vinegar, mustard, garlic and black pepper. Slowly drizzle in olive oil, whisking until smooth and well blended. Taste, and adjust seasonings.

Guacamole Salad

Makes 4 side-dish servings • Each serving: 4 grams protein • 9 grams carbohydrate

2 ripe avocados

1 tablespoon fresh lemon juice

1 seeded and chopped large, ripe tomato

1 minced garlic clove

1 tablespoon chopped red onion

1 tablespoon chopped fresh cilantro

1 small minced fresh jalapeño pepper (optional), or *1 to 2 tablespoons canned diced green chilies, to taste* [wear rubber gloves to prepare fresh jalapeño pepper]

freshly ground black pepper, to taste

dash hot-pepper sauce

4 cups mixed salad greens

Cut avocados in half. Remove pits and scoop flesh into a medium bowl. Using a fork, mash avocado with lemon juice.

To seed tomato, cut tomato in half and squeeze gently. Scoop out seeds with a small spoon or your fingers and chop tomato. To mashed avocados, gently mix in tomato, garlic, onion, cilantro, jalapeño pepper, black pepper and hot-pepper sauce. Taste, and adjust seasonings. Serve on a bed of mixed salad greens.

Mixed-Greens Salad

Makes 4 side-dish servings • Each serving: 4 grams protein • 4 grams carbohydrate

4 cups mixed salad greens

Optional Additions

½ cup diced cucumbers

½ cup sliced radishes

1 cup shredded red cabbage

1 cup shredded radicchio

½ cup diced celery stalks

*1 cup sliced brown or white
mushrooms*

½ cup grated carrots

*1 cup thinly sliced red or green
bell peppers*

½ cup thinly sliced fennel

½ cup diced scallions

½ cup thinly sliced red onion

¼ cup raw sunflower seeds

¼ cup diced raw walnuts

In a large bowl, toss ingredients with your choice of dressing. (See Salad Dressings, starting on page 149.)

Mixed-Greens Salad with Chèvre (Goat Cheese)

Makes 4 side-dish servings • Each serving: 7 grams protein • trace carbohydrate

4 (¾-inch) rounds of chèvre (goat cheese) cut from a log of chèvre

¼ cup pure-pressed extra virgin olive oil

Classic Salad Dressing

2 teaspoons mixed dried Italian herbs (oregano, basil, marjoram, thyme)

4 cups mixed salad greens

Place goat cheese rounds in a shallow baking dish. Combine olive oil and herbs and pour over cheese. Marinate several hours or overnight, covered, in refrigerator.

Preheat oven to 375°. Bake cheese 15 minutes or until softened.

Wash and dry greens. Arrange salad greens on individual plates. Place a round of baked goat cheese in center of each plate on top of salad greens. Drizzle Classic Salad Dressing over salad greens and serve immediately.

Classic Salad Dressing

½ cup balsamic vinegar

½ cup pure-pressed extra virgin olive oil

freshly ground black pepper, to taste

In a small bowl, using a fork, whisk vinegar, olive oil and black pepper until smooth.

Mixed-Greens Salad with Toasted Walnuts and Gorgonzola Cheese

Makes 4 side-dish servings • Each serving: 9 grams protein • 3 grams carbohydrate

½ cup chopped raw walnuts

4 cups mixed salad greens

Dijon Vinaigrette

½ cup crumbled Gorgonzola cheese

Put walnuts in an ungreased skillet over medium-high heat. Stir nuts or shake pan almost constantly until walnuts are evenly browned and toasted. Remove from pan immediately and set aside.

In a large bowl, toss salad greens with Dijon Vinaigrette. Sprinkle with toasted walnuts and Gorgonzola cheese.

Dijon Vinaigrette

1 minced garlic clove

2 tablespoons Dijon mustard

¼ cup balsamic vinegar

½ cup pure-pressed extra virgin olive oil

freshly ground black pepper, to taste

In a blender or food processor, combine all ingredients and blend until smooth; or place ingredients in a jar with a tight-fitting lid and shake vigorously until well blended. Taste, and adjust seasonings.

Mushroom and Artichoke Salad

Makes 4 side-dish servings • Each serving: 3 grams protein • 7 grams carbohydrate

1 pound brown or white
   mushrooms, stems removed
   and thickly sliced
1 cup marinated artichoke
   hearts, drained and quartered

4 chopped celery stalks
¼ cup chopped fresh parsley
½ thinly sliced red onion
Mushroom Marinade

Combine mushrooms, artichoke hearts, celery, parsley and onion. Pour Mushroom Marinade over salad. Refrigerate and marinate 30 minutes before serving.

Mushroom Marinade

3 tablespoons red wine vinegar
1½ tablespoons chopped fresh
   tarragon, or 1 teaspoon dried
   tarragon

freshly ground black pepper,
   to taste
¼ cup pure-pressed extra virgin
   olive oil

In a small bowl, using a fork, whisk vinegar, tarragon and black pepper. Slowly drizzle in olive oil, whisking constantly until smooth. Taste, and adjust seasonings.

Pear and Gorgonzola Winter Salad

Makes 4 side-dish servings • Each serving: 9 grams protein • 10 grams carbohydrate

½ cup chopped raw walnuts

1 large head butter lettuce, washed, dried and torn into bite-size pieces

2 cored and sliced ripe pears

½ cup crumbled Gorgonzola cheese

2 tablespoons chopped fresh parsley

Winter Vinaigrette

Put walnuts in an ungreased skillet over medium-high heat. Stir nuts or shake pan almost constantly until walnuts are evenly browned and toasted. Remove from pan immediately and set aside.

Line 4 individual plates with washed and dried lettuce. Arrange pears on top. Sprinkle with Gorgonzola cheese, toasted walnuts and parsley. Spoon on Winter Vinaigrette.

Winter Vinaigrette

2 tablespoons raspberry vinegar

4 tablespoons pure-pressed extra virgin olive oil

freshly ground black pepper, to taste

In a small bowl, using a fork, whisk vinegar, olive oil and black pepper until smooth.

Picnic Potato Salad

Makes 6 side-dish servings • Each serving: 7 grams protein • 8 grams carbohydrate

5 medium red potatoes (peeled, if desired)

2 diced celery stalks

1 small diced red onion

2 tablespoons chopped fresh parsley

3 peeled and diced hard-boiled eggs (optional)*

1 diced red bell pepper

8 green beans, ends trimmed, sliced diagonally into 1-inch pieces and steamed until tender

Picnic Potato Salad Dressing

Boil potatoes until just barely tender, about 10 to 15 minutes. Drain and let cool. Toss potatoes and all other ingredients with Picnic Potato Salad Dressing until well coated.

Picnic Potato Salad Dressing

2 tablespoons fresh lemon juice

1 tablespoon Dijon mustard

1 egg yolk (optional)**

1 minced garlic clove

freshly ground black pepper, to taste

¼ cup pure-pressed extra virgin olive oil

2 tablespoons minced fresh chives

In a small bowl, using a fork, whisk lemon juice, mustard, egg yolk, garlic and black pepper. Slowly drizzle in oil, whisking continuously. Add chives and stir until well blended. Taste, and adjust seasonings.

---

*To hard boil eggs, place eggs in a saucepan and cover with cold water. Bring to a boil uncovered. Allow to boil for 1 minute, then cover, remove from heat and let sit undisturbed 10 minutes. Rinse eggs under cold water. Crack shells, peel and rinse eggs.

**If you are concerned about using raw egg, omit the egg yolk from this recipe.

Red Cabbage with Walnuts Salad

Makes 4 side-dish servings • Each serving: 5 grams protein • 3 grams carbohydrate

1 small coarsely shredded red
  cabbage
½ cup diced walnuts

2 tablespoons chopped fresh mint
Red Cabbage Vinaigrette

Combine red cabbage, walnuts and fresh mint. Toss with Red Cabbage Vinaigrette and marinate 30 minutes, refrigerated, before serving.

Red Cabbage Vinaigrette

3 tablespoons red wine vinegar
2 teaspoons Dijon mustard
freshly ground black pepper,
  to taste

½ cup pure-pressed extra virgin
  olive oil

In a small bowl, using a fork, whisk vinegar, mustard and black pepper. Slowly drizzle in olive oil, whisking constantly until smooth.

Roasted Potato, Asparagus, Red Pepper and Feta Cheese Salad

Makes 6 side-dish servings • Each serving: 8 grams protein • 25 grams carbohydrate

2 pounds red potatoes (peeled, if desired)

2 tablespoons pure-pressed extra virgin olive oil

2 minced garlic cloves

freshly ground black pepper, to taste

3 red bell peppers, roasted, or ¾ cup store-bought roasted red bell peppers

1 pound asparagus (tough ends trimmed), sliced diagonally into 1-inch pieces

1 cup diced celery stalks

½ cup slivered fresh basil, or 2 teaspoons dried basil, or ¼ cup minced fresh parsley

½ cup crumbled feta cheese

Roasted Salad Dressing (see recipe, page 140)

4 cups mixed salad greens

Preheat oven to 400°. Cut potatoes into 1-inch cubes. Toss with olive oil, garlic and black pepper. Spread potatoes evenly over a lightly greased baking sheet. Roast until browned and tender, about 20 to 30 minutes, turning occasionally. Set aside.

If using fresh red bell peppers, roast peppers directly over a gas flame or under a preheated broiler on a broiler rack. Using tongs, turn peppers frequently until blistered and blackened on all sides. Place peppers in a bowl with a plate on top. Let steam for 15 minutes to loosen skins. Peel off all charred skin. Discard skin along with seeds. Cut roasted flesh into slivers. Set aside.

Cook asparagus until just barely tender by immersing into boiling water about 3 to 6 minutes. Drain, rinse under cold water and drain again.

Gently toss roasted potatoes with bell peppers, asparagus and celery. Add fresh basil or parsley and crumbled feta cheese. Toss with Roasted Salad Dressing. Serve on a bed of salad greens.

Roasted Salad Dressing

2 tablespoons balsamic vinegar

2 teaspoons Dijon mustard

1 minced garlic clove

freshly ground black pepper,
*   to taste*

4 tablespoons pure-pressed extra
*   virgin olive oil*

In a small bowl, using a fork, whisk vinegar, mustard, garlic and black pepper. Slowly drizzle in olive oil and continue whisking until smooth and well blended.

Roasted Vegetable Salad

Makes 4 side-dish servings • Each serving: 3 grams protein • 15 grams carbohydrate

1 large sweet potato, peeled and chopped into 1-inch cubes

1 cup green beans, ends trimmed, sliced diagonally into 1-inch pieces

1 tablespoon pure-pressed extra virgin olive oil

freshly ground black pepper, to taste

1 coarsely chopped red onion

1 red bell pepper, chopped into large chunks

1 tablespoon pure-pressed extra virgin olive oil

8 ounces brown or white mushrooms, stemmed and left whole

2 medium zucchini, sliced into ¼-inch rounds

1 tablespoon pure-pressed extra virgin olive oil

¼ cup balsamic vinegar

2 teaspoons Dijon mustard

¼ cup slivered fresh basil or minced parsley, for garnish

Preheat oven to 400°. Combine sweet potatoes and green beans with 1 tablespoon olive oil and black pepper. Arrange on a lightly greased baking sheet and roast, turning occasionally.

In a medium bowl, toss red onion and bell pepper with 1 tablespoon olive oil and black pepper. When sweet potatoes and beans have roasted for about 10 minutes, remove baking sheet from oven and add onion and pepper mixture, stirring well to mix. Return to oven.

While potato, bean, onion and pepper combination is roasting, combine mushrooms and zucchini and mix with 1 tablespoon olive oil and black pepper. When potato, bean, onion and pepper combination has roasted together for 5 to 10 minutes, add mushroom and zucchini mixture, stirring well to mix. Roast all together for about 5 to 10 minutes until vegetables are nicely browned and tender. Remove from oven.

In a medium serving bowl, toss all roasted vegetables with balsamic vinegar mixed with mustard. Sprinkle with slivered fresh basil or parsley. Serve at room temperature.

Russian Vegetable Salad

Makes 6 side-dish servings • Each serving: 4 grams protein • 8 grams carbohydrate

4 golden or red beets	*2 diced carrots*
2 large red potatoes (peeled, if desired)	*2 tablespoons minced fresh parsley*
½ pound green beans, ends trimmed, and sliced diagonally into 1-inch pieces	*3 tablespoons drained and rinsed capers*
	Russian Vinaigrette

Boil whole beets in water to cover until tender, about 35 to 40 minutes. Drain and cool. Peel and dice into small cubes. Boil whole potatoes in water to cover until tender, about 25 to 30 minutes. Drain and cool. Dice into small cubes. Cook green beans and carrots in boiling water until tender, about 10 to 15 minutes. Drain and rinse under cold water.

In a large bowl, toss beets, potatoes, green beans, carrots, parsley and capers with Russian Vinaigrette.

Russian Vinaigrette

3 tablespoons balsamic vinegar	*3 tablespoons pure-pressed extra virgin olive oil*
1 tablespoon Dijon mustard	
freshly ground black pepper, to taste	

In a small bowl, using a fork, whisk balsamic vinegar, mustard and black pepper. Slowly drizzle in olive oil, whisking constantly until smooth. Pour over diced vegetables and toss gently.

Seattle Caesar Salad

Makes 4 side-dish servings • Each serving: 5 grams protein • trace carbohydrate

1 head romaine lettuce, washed, patted dry and torn into large pieces

Seattle Caesar Dressing

In a large serving bowl, toss washed and dried lettuce with Seattle Caesar Dressing. Serve immediately on chilled salad plates.

Seattle Caesar Dressing

2 minced garlic cloves

2 tablespoons fresh lemon juice

1 tablespoon balsamic vinegar

¼ cup pure-pressed extra virgin olive oil

1 teaspoon Dijon mustard

1 egg yolk (optional)*

6 tablespoons grated Parmesan cheese

freshly ground black pepper, to taste

In a blender or food processor, combine all ingredients until smooth. Taste, and adjust seasonings. Store covered in refrigerator.

———————

*If you are concerned about using raw eggs, omit the egg yolk from this recipe.

Spinach Salad with Avocado and Mushrooms

Makes 4 side-dish servings • Each serving: 7 grams protein • 8 grams carbohydrate

1 pound fresh spinach leaves, washed, dried and torn into bite-size pieces

2 ripe avocados, peeled, diced and sprinkled with the juice of a ½ of a fresh lemon

8 ounces thinly sliced brown or white mushrooms

¼ cup diced scallions

Garlic Dijon Vinaigrette

In a large serving bowl, toss all ingredients gently with Garlic Dijon Vinaigrette and serve immediately.

Garlic Dijon Vinaigrette

3 tablespoons balsamic vinegar

2 minced garlic cloves

1 tablespoon Dijon mustard

1 tablespoon slivered fresh basil, or 1 teaspoon dried basil

¾ cup pure-pressed extra virgin olive oil

freshly ground black pepper, to taste

In a blender or food processor, combine all ingredients and blend until smooth; or place ingredients in a jar with a tight-fitting lid and shake vigorously until well blended. Taste, and adjust seasonings.

Tabouli Salad

Makes 4 side-dish servings • Each serving: 8 grams protein • 24 grams carbohydrate

¾ cup bulgur wheat

1 ½ cups water

4 cups finely chopped fresh
  parsley

1 bunch finely chopped scallions

1 large bunch finely chopped
  fresh mint

3 medium chopped tomatoes

½ cup fresh lemon juice

½ cup pure-pressed extra virgin
  olive oil

freshly ground black pepper,
  to taste

1 head romaine lettuce, washed
  and patted dry

Pour bulgur into a bowl and cover with water. Let sit 20 minutes. Drain well, squeezing out extra water through a fine strainer or cloth. Combine drained bulgur with parsley, scallions, mint, tomatoes, lemon juice, olive oil and black pepper. Taste, and adjust seasonings.

Arrange washed and dried romaine leaves on individual plates and mound with tabouli salad.

Tofu "Egg" Salad

Makes 4 side-dish servings • Each serving: 9 grams protein • trace carbohydrate

1 pound firm tofu, drained, pressed and crumbled (for directions, see "All You Need to Know About Tofu," page 10)

⅓ cup mayonnaise (made from pure-pressed oil)

1 tablespoon Dijon mustard

½ cup minced celery stalks

2 teaspoons fresh lemon or lime juice

1 teaspoon dried dill

2 tablespoons minced scallions

2 tablespoons minced fresh parsley

1 tablespoon drained and rinsed capers (optional)

1½ teaspoons ground turmeric

freshly ground black pepper, to taste

dash cayenne pepper

In a small bowl, using a fork, mix all ingredients until well blended. Taste, and adjust seasonings. Refrigerate 1 hour before serving.

Salad Dressings

We care about your opinions. Please take a moment to fill out this Reader Survey card and mail it back to us. As a special **"thank you"** we'll send you exciting news about interesting books and a valuable **Gift Certificate.**

Please PRINT using ALL CAPS

Name First _____ MI. ☐ Last Name _____

Address _____

City _____ ST ☐ Zip _____

Phone # (☐) _____ Fax # (☐) _____

Email _____

(1) Gender:
_____ Female _____ Male

(2) Age:
1) _____ 12 or under
2) _____ 13-19
3) _____ 20-39
4) _____ 40-59
5) _____ 60+

(3) Marital Status
_____ Married
_____ Single
_____ Divorced/Widowed

(4) Did you receive this book as a gift?
_____ Yes _____ No

(5) How many Health Communications books have you bought or read?
_____ 1 _____ 2-4 _____ 5+

(6) How did you find out about this book?
Please fill in ONE.
1) _____ Recommendation
2) _____ Store Display
3) _____ Bestseller List
4) _____ Online
5) _____ Advertisement
6) _____ Catalog/Mailing
7) _____ Interview/Review (TV, Radio, Print)

(7) Where do you usually buy books?
Please fill in your top TWO choices.
1) _____ Bookstore
2) _____ Religious Bookstore
3) _____ Online
4) _____ Book Club/Mail Order
5) _____ Price Club (Costco, Sam's Club, etc.)
6) _____ Retail Store (Target, Wal-Mart, etc.)

(9) What subjects do you enjoy reading about most? Rank only *FIVE. Use 1 for your favorite, 2 for second favorite, etc.*

	1	2	3	4	5
1) Parenting/Family	○	○	○	○	○
2) Relationships	○	○	○	○	○
3) Recovery/Addictions	○	○	○	○	○
4) Health/Nutrition	○	○	○	○	○
5) Christianity	○	○	○	○	○
6) Spirituality/Inspiration	○	○	○	○	○
7) Business Self-Help	○	○	○	○	○
8) Teen Issues	○	○	○	○	○
9) Sports	○	○	○	○	○

(14) What attracts you most to a book?
(Please rank 1-4 in order of preference.)

	1	2	3	4
1) Title	○	○	○	○
2) Cover Design	○	○	○	○
3) Author	○	○	○	○
4) Content	○	○	○	○

TAPE IN MIDDLE; DO NOT STAPLE

BUSINESS REPLY MAIL
FIRST-CLASS MAIL PERMIT NO 45 DEERFIELD BEACH, FL

POSTAGE WILL BE PAID BY ADDRESSEE

THE SCHWARZBEIN PRINCIPLE
3201 SW 15TH STREET
DEERFIELD BEACH FL 33442-9875

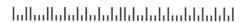

FOLD HERE

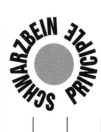

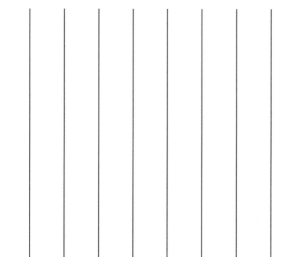

Comments:

Asian Citrus Dressing

Makes about 1 cup • 1 tablespoon: trace protein • trace carbohydrate

Use on spinach or mixed-greens salads.

1 minced garlic clove

1 teaspoon peeled and finely minced fresh ginger

2 tablespoons minced scallions

2 tablespoons fresh lime juice

2 tablespoons fresh orange juice

1 tablespoon rice wine vinegar

2 teaspoons low-sodium tamari soy sauce

¼ cup pure-pressed peanut oil

¼ cup pure-pressed sesame oil

dash cayenne pepper

In a blender or food processor, combine all ingredients and blend until smooth; or place ingredients in a jar with a tight-fitting lid and shake vigorously until well blended. Taste, and adjust seasonings. Store covered in refrigerator. Bring to room temperature before using.

Balsamic Vinaigrette

Makes about 1 cup • 1 tablespoon: trace protein • trace carbohydrate

Use on mixed-greens, spinach, marinated or roasted vegetable salads.

¼ cup balsamic vinegar

2 tablespoons fresh lemon juice

1 tablespoon Dijon mustard

2 minced garlic cloves

½ cup pure-pressed extra virgin olive oil

freshly ground black pepper, to taste

In a blender or food processor, combine all ingredients and blend until smooth; or place ingredients in a jar with a tight-fitting lid and shake vigorously until well blended. Taste, and adjust seasonings. Store covered in refrigerator. Bring to room temperature before using.

Bleu Cheese Dressing

Makes about 2 cups • 1 tablespoon: 1 gram protein • trace carbohydrate

Use on spinach, mixed-greens or potato salads.

½ cup whole sour cream

½ cup mayonnaise (made from pure-pressed oil)

⅔ cup crumbled bleu cheese

1 minced garlic clove

2 tablespoons fresh lemon juice

2 teaspoons dried basil

freshly ground black pepper, to taste

In a blender or food processor, combine all ingredients and blend until smooth; or place ingredients in a jar with a tight-fitting lid and shake vigorously until well blended. Taste, and adjust seasonings. Cover and refrigerate several hours before using.

Caesar Dressing

Makes about ¾ cup • 1 tablespoon: 2 grams protein • trace carbohydrate

Use on romaine lettuce or potato salads.

2 minced garlic cloves

2 tablespoons fresh lemon juice

1 tablespoon balsamic vinegar

¼ cup pure-pressed extra virgin olive oil

1 teaspoon Dijon mustard

1 egg yolk (optional)*

6 tablespoons grated Parmesan cheese

freshly ground black pepper, to taste

In a blender or food processor, combine all ingredients and blend until smooth. Taste, and adjust seasonings. Store covered in refrigerator.

---

*If you are concerned about using raw egg, omit the egg yolk from this recipe.

Chèvre (Goat Cheese) Dressing

Makes about 1½ cups • 1 tablespoon: 1 gram protein • trace carbohydrate

Use on roasted vegetable, mixed-greens, spinach or potato salads.

½ cup crumbled chèvre (goat
  cheese)

1 cup all-dairy heavy cream

1 teaspoon Dijon mustard

2 tablespoons finely chopped
  shallots

2 tablespoons finely slivered
  fresh basil, or 1 teaspoon dried
  basil

freshly ground black pepper,
  to taste

In a medium bowl, using a fork, whisk all ingredients until smooth and well blended. Taste, and adjust seasonings. Store covered in refrigerator.

Creamy Dill Dressing

Makes about 1 cup • 1 tablespoon: trace protein • trace carbohydrate

Use on mixed-greens, spinach, marinated or roasted vegetable or potato salads.

½ cup mayonnaise (made from
  pure-pressed oil)

½ cup whole sour cream

1 teaspoon red wine vinegar

1 tablespoon fresh lime juice

1 tablespoon minced fresh parsley

1 tablespoon minced scallions

1 tablespoon minced fresh dill, or
  1 teaspoon dried dill

freshly ground black pepper,
  to taste

In a medium bowl, using a fork, whisk all ingredients until smooth. Taste, and adjust seasonings. Chill before using.

Creamy Vinaigrette

Makes about 1³/₄ cups • 1 tablespoon: trace protein • trace carbohydrate

Use on mixed-greens, marinated vegetable, spinach or potato salads.

½ cup red wine vinegar

2 tablespoons Dijon mustard

2 tablespoons fresh lemon juice

1 minced garlic clove

1 to 2 teaspoons peeled and finely minced fresh ginger (optional)

1 cup pure-pressed extra virgin olive oil

freshly ground black pepper, to taste

In a blender or food processor, combine all ingredients and blend until smooth; or place ingredients in a jar with a tight-fitting lid, and shake vigorously until well blended. Taste, and adjust seasonings. Store covered in refrigerator. Bring to room temperature before using.

French Dressing

Makes about 1½ cups • 1 tablespoon: trace protein • trace carbohydrate

Use on mixed-greens salads or marinated vegetable salads.

½ cup red wine vinegar

2 minced garlic cloves

½ teaspoon dried oregano

½ teaspoon dried basil

1 teaspoon dried tarragon

1 tablespoon Dijon mustard

freshly ground black pepper, to taste

1 cup pure-pressed extra virgin olive oil

In a small bowl, using a fork, whisk all ingredients, except olive oil. Slowly drizzle in olive oil, whisking constantly until dressing is well blended. Taste, and adjust seasonings. Store covered in refrigerator. Bring to room temperature before using.

French Vinaigrette with Feta Cheese

Makes about 1 cup • 1 tablespoon: 1 gram protein • trace carbohydrate

Use on mixed-greens or spinach salads.

⅓ cup red wine vinegar

1 tablespoon Dijon mustard

⅓ cup pure-pressed extra virgin
  olive oil

1 tablespoon minced fresh parsley

freshly ground black pepper,
  to taste

⅓ cup crumbled feta cheese

In a small bowl, using a fork, whisk red wine vinegar and mustard. Slowly drizzle in olive oil, whisking constantly until vinaigrette thickens. Stir in parsley, black pepper and feta cheese. Taste, and adjust seasonings. Store covered in refrigerator. Bring to room temperature before using.

Garlic Vinaigrette

Makes about 1³/₄ cup • 1 tablespoon: trace protein • trace carbohydrate

Use on mixed-greens, spinach, roasted or marinated vegetable salads, or coleslaws.

5 minced garlic cloves

2 tablespoons Dijon mustard

½ cup red wine vinegar

1 cup pure-pressed extra virgin
  olive oil

¼ cup finely chopped fresh parsley

freshly ground black pepper,
  to taste

In a small bowl, using a fork, whisk garlic, mustard and vinegar until well blended. Slowly drizzle in olive oil in a steady stream, whisking until well blended. Stir in parsley and black pepper. Taste, and adjust seasonings. Store covered in refrigerator. Bring to room temperature before using.

Green Goddess Dressing

Makes about 1⅓ cups • 1 tablespoon: trace protein • trace carbohydrate

Use on mixed-greens, mixed-vegetable or potato salads.

½ cup mayonnaise (made from
  pure-pressed oil)

½ cup whole sour cream

3 tablespoons all-dairy heavy
  cream

1 tablespoon tarragon wine
  vinegar

2 teaspoons fresh lemon juice

1 minced garlic clove

¼ cup finely chopped fresh parsley

2 tablespoons thinly sliced scallions

2 tablespoons minced fresh chives

2 tablespoons finely chopped
  fresh tarragon leaves, or
  2 teaspoons dried tarragon

freshly ground black pepper,
  to taste

In a blender or food processor, combine all ingredients and blend until smooth; or place ingredients in a jar with a tight-fitting lid and shake vigorously until well blended. Taste, and adjust seasonings. Store covered in refrigerator.

Healing Oil Dressing

Makes about 1¹/₂ cups • 1 tablespoon: trace protein • trace carbohydrate

Use on mixed-greens or mixed-vegetable salads.

⅓ cup pure-pressed safflower oil

⅓ cup pure-pressed extra virgin olive oil

⅓ cup pure-pressed flaxseed oil

2 minced garlic cloves

1½ tablespoons Dijon mustard

⅓ cup balsamic vinegar

In a blender or food processor, combine all ingredients and blend until smooth; or place ingredients in a jar with a tight-fitting lid and shake vigorously until well blended. Taste, and adjust seasonings. Store covered in refrigerator. Bring to room temperature before using.

Middle Eastern Dressing

Makes about ³/₄ cup • 1 tablespoon: trace protein • trace carbohydrate

Use on mixed-vegetable, carrot or spinach salads, or coleslaws.

½ cup pure-pressed extra virgin olive oil

¼ cup fresh lemon or lime juice

1 minced garlic clove

1 teaspoon grated lemon or lime zest

2 tablespoons chopped fresh parsley

1 tablespoon minced scallions

1 teaspoon ground cumin

¼ teaspoon dried mustard

dash cayenne pepper

In a blender or food processor, combine all ingredients and blend until smooth; or place ingredients in a jar with a tight-fitting lid, and shake vigorously until well blended. Taste, and adjust seasonings. Store covered in refrigerator. Bring to room temperature before using.

Oriental Vinaigrette

Makes about 1 cup • 1 tablespoon: trace protein • trace carbohydrate

Use on vegetable salads.

¼ cup fresh lime juice

2 teaspoons grated lime zest

2 minced garlic cloves

4 teaspoons peeled and finely
   minced fresh ginger

¼ cup rice wine vinegar

4 teaspoons low-sodium tamari
   soy sauce

2 teaspoons Dijon mustard

cayenne pepper, to taste

¼ cup pure-pressed peanut oil

¼ cup pure-pressed sesame oil

In a small bowl, using a fork, whisk lime juice, lime zest, garlic, ginger, vinegar, soy sauce, mustard and cayenne pepper. Slowly whisk in peanut and sesame oils until well blended. Taste, and adjust seasonings. Store covered in refrigerator. Bring to room temperature before using.

Parmesan Salad Dressing

Makes about 1½ cups • 1 tablespoon: 1 gram protein • trace carbohydrate

Use on mixed-greens, spinach, mushroom or mixed-greens salads.

½ cup fresh lemon juice

¾ cup pure-pressed extra virgin
   olive oil

1 tablespoon Dijon mustard

¼ cup grated Parmesan cheese

1 teaspoon dried basil

1 tablespoon chopped scallions

freshly ground black pepper,
   to taste

In a blender or food processor, combine all ingredients and blend until smooth; or place ingredients in a jar with a tight-fitting lid and shake vigorously until well blended. Taste, and adjust seasonings. Store covered in refrigerator. Bring to room temperature before using.

Ranch-Style Dressing

Makes about 1 cup • 1 tablespoon: trace protein • trace carbohydrate

Use on mixed-greens or spinach salads, or on baked potatoes.

½ cup mayonnaise (made from
   pure-pressed oil)

½ cup whole sour cream

1 minced garlic clove

1 teaspoon Dijon mustard

½ teaspoon dried dill

freshly ground black pepper,
   to taste

In a blender or food processor, combine all ingredients and blend until smooth; or place ingredients in a jar with a tight-fitting lid, and shake vigorously until well blended. Cover and refrigerate several hours before using. Taste, and adjust seasonings. Store covered in refrigerator.

Sun-Dried Tomato Vinaigrette

Makes about 1¼ cups • 1 tablespoon: trace protein • 1 gram carbohydrate

Use on mixed-greens, spinach or roasted vegetable salads.

¼ cup sun-dried tomatoes
  packed in olive oil

½ cup pure-pressed extra virgin
  olive oil

⅓ cup balsamic vinegar

2 tablespoons fresh lemon juice

2 minced garlic cloves

¼ cup slivered fresh basil, or
  2 teaspoons dried basil

2 teaspoons Dijon mustard

freshly ground black pepper,
  to taste

In a blender or food processor, combine all ingredients and blend until smooth; or place ingredients in a jar with a tight-fitting lid and shake vigorously until well blended. Add 2 to 4 tablespoons water to thin, if desired. Store covered in refrigerator. Bring to room temperature before using.

Tahini Dressing

Makes about 1 cup • 1 tablespoon: 2 grams protein • 1 gram carbohydrate

Use on mixed-greens or spinach salads.

¼ pound well-drained firm tofu, cubed (for directions, see "All You Need to Know About Tofu," page 10)

¼ cup pure-pressed vegetable oil

1 minced garlic clove

2 tablespoons fresh lemon juice

2 tablespoons sesame tahini

1 tablespoon low-sodium tamari soy sauce

1 tablespoon chopped scallions

freshly ground black pepper, to taste

2 tablespoons vegetable stock (see recipe, page 100), or low-sodium canned or water, to thin (optional)

In a blender or food processor, combine all ingredients except vegetable stock or water and blend until smooth. Thin with stock or water if desired. Taste, and adjust seasonings. Store covered in refrigerator.

Thai Vinaigrette

Makes about ³/₄ cup • 1 tablespoon: trace protein • trace carbohydrate

Use on mixed-greens, spinach or marinated-vegetable salads.

2 tablespoons fresh lime juice

2 tablespoons rice wine vinegar

1 tablespoon low-sodium tamari soy sauce

1 minced garlic clove

2 tablespoons minced fresh mint

2 tablespoons slivered fresh basil

2 tablespoons minced fresh cilantro

2 teaspoons peeled and finely minced fresh ginger

1 tablespoon hot chili oil

¼ cup pure-pressed extra virgin olive oil

¼ teaspoon red-pepper flakes (optional)

In a blender or food processor, combine all ingredients and blend until smooth; or place ingredients in a jar with a tight-fitting lid and shake vigorously until well blended. Taste, and adjust seasonings. Cover and refrigerate several hours before using. Store covered in refrigerator.

Thousand Island Dressing

Makes about 1 ²/₃ cups • 1 tablespoon: trace protein • trace carbohydrate

Use on mixed-greens or spinach salads.

1 cup mayonnaise (made from pure-pressed oil)

¼ cup chili sauce, or tomato sauce

¼ cup whole plain yogurt

2 tablespoons minced dill pickles

1 chopped hard-boiled egg*

1 tablespoon finely chopped scallions

1 tablespoon finely chopped fresh parsley

freshly ground black pepper, to taste

In a medium bowl, using a fork, combine all ingredients until well blended and smooth. Taste, and adjust seasonings. Store covered in refrigerator.

---

*To hard boil eggs, place eggs in a saucepan and cover with cold water. Bring to a boil uncovered. Allow to boil for 1 minute, then cover, remove from heat and let sit undisturbed 10 minutes. Rinse eggs under cold water. Crack shells, peel and rinse eggs.

Vegetarian Entrées

Asian Mint Pesto Tofu Kabobs

Makes 4 servings • Each serving: 34 grams protein • 3 grams carbohydrate

1¼ cups Asian Mint Pesto

1½ pounds firm tofu, drained, pressed and cut into 1½-inch pieces (for directions, see "All You Need to Know About Tofu," page 10)

16 brown or white mushrooms, wiped clean with a damp cloth

2 red bell peppers, cut into 1-inch squares

eight 8-inch bamboo skewers soaked in water 15 minutes to prevent burning

Asian Mint Pesto

2 cups loosely packed fresh mint leaves

½ cup loosely packed fresh basil leaves

½ cup loosely packed fresh cilantro

½ cup grated Parmesan cheese

2 minced garlic cloves

2 tablespoons fresh lime juice

½ cup pure-pressed extra virgin olive oil

freshly ground black pepper, to taste

In a food processor, combine all pesto ingredients until well blended. Taste, and adjust seasonings. Coat tofu pieces with pesto paste and refrigerate at least 30 minutes, or overnight if possible.

Preheat oven to 400°. Thread 3 to 5 chunks of tofu onto each skewer, alternating with mushrooms and red bell peppers. Place skewers on a greased rack with a tinfoil-lined baking sheet underneath. Bake until tofu is evenly browned, turning occasionally, about 20 minutes.

Tofu skewers can also be grilled on a barbecue. Turn occasionally until browned, about 15 minutes.

Baked Chili Rellenos

Makes 6 servings • Each serving: 22 grams protein • 3 grams carbohydrate
(Nutritional information does not include salsa)

8 fresh pasilla chilies, or
8 canned whole green chilies
[wear rubber gloves to
prepare fresh chili pepper]

2 cups whole cottage cheese

*1½ cups grated Monterey Jack
cheese*

1 teaspoon dried oregano

dash cayenne pepper

4 eggs

½ cup all-dairy heavy cream

½ cup water

*freshly ground black pepper,
to taste*

¼ teaspoon garlic powder

*2 tablespoons minced fresh
cilantro, for garnish*

*2 tablespoons minced scallions,
for garnish*

*1 cup salsa (see Salsas, starting
on page 296),* or *store-bought*

If using fresh pasilla chilies, roast pasilla chili peppers directly over a gas flame or under preheated broiler on a broiler rack. Using tongs, turn peppers frequently until blistered and blackened on all sides. Place peppers in a bowl with a plate on top. Let steam for 15 minutes to loosen skins. Peel off all charred skin. Discard skin along with seeds. Cut roasted flesh into thick strips.

Preheat oven to 375°. Lightly oil a 10-inch pie pan. Arrange chilies in a single layer on bottom of pan. In a medium bowl, using a fork, mix cottage cheese, grated cheese, oregano and cayenne pepper. Spread mixture smoothly over chilies.

In a medium bowl, whisk eggs, cream, water, black pepper and garlic powder. Pour over chili and cheese layers.

Bake 30 to 35 minutes until puffed, firm and golden brown. Sprinkle top with minced cilantro and scallions. Serve with salsa on the side.

Baked Stuffed Green Peppers

Makes 6 servings • Each serving: 16 grams protein • 33 grams carbohydrate

6 large green bell peppers

4 cups cooked brown rice

1½ cups grated Monterey Jack cheese

½ cup minced fresh parsley

½ cup minced scallions

½ cup chopped raw pecans or raw walnuts

1 tablespoon Dijon mustard

2 beaten eggs

freshly ground black pepper, to taste

dash cayenne pepper

Preheat oven to 350°. Slice tops from green peppers and remove seeds. In a large skillet, bring 2 cups of water to a boil. Add peppers, reduce heat to low and simmer until just tender, about 5 minutes. Remove from pan, drain and set aside to cool.

In a medium bowl, combine rice, cheese, parsley, scallions, pecans or walnuts, mustard, eggs, black pepper and cayenne pepper. Spoon rice mixture into peppers.

Arrange filled peppers in a shallow baking dish. Add water to a ¼-inch depth in dish to prevent burning. Bake 30 to 35 minutes until filling is hot.

Place under broiler briefly to brown.

Black Bean and Goat Cheese Enchiladas

Makes 8 servings • Each serving: 18 grams protein • 44 grams carbohydrate

Red Sauce

2 tablespoons pure-pressed extra
  virgin olive oil

1 large diced onion

2 minced garlic cloves

½ teaspoon ground cumin

1 teaspoon dried oregano

28 ounces canned enchilada
  sauce

¼ cup tomato paste

freshly ground black pepper,
  to taste

In a large nonstick skillet, heat oil over medium-high heat. When oil is hot, add onion, garlic, cumin and oregano and sauté until softened, about 5 minutes. Add canned enchilada sauce, tomato paste and black pepper. Bring to a boil, reduce heat to low and simmer 15 minutes, stirring occasionally.

Enchilada Filling

1½ cups cooked, drained black
  beans

1 mango, diced

½ cup diced scallions

2 tablespoons minced fresh
  cilantro

½ cup fresh corn kernels
  or frozen and thawed

1 cup crumbled chèvre
  (goat cheese)

1½ cups whole cottage cheese

1 tablespoon fresh lime juice

2 teaspoons chili powder

freshly ground black pepper,
  to taste

12 corn tortillas

2 tablespoons minced scallions,
  for garnish

1 tablespoon minced fresh
  cilantro, for garnish

In a large bowl, using a fork, blend cooked beans, mango, scallions, cilantro, corn, chèvre (goat cheese), cottage cheese, lime juice, chili powder and black pepper. Taste, and adjust seasonings.

Preheat oven to 350°. Pour 1 cup enchilada sauce into a 9×13-inch baking dish. Dip tortillas, one at a time, in simmering enchilada sauce in skillet, about 5 seconds to soften, thoroughly coating both sides. Using tongs, transfer each tortilla to a plate. Spoon about ¼ cup filling on each tortilla, just off center. Roll tortilla around filling and place seam-side down in baking pan. Repeat with remaining tortillas.

Spread remaining sauce over filled tortillas. Bake, uncovered, 25 minutes until hot and bubbly. Sprinkle with minced scallions and cilantro.

Black Bean Chili

Makes 8 servings • Each serving: 10 grams protein • 18 grams carbohydrate

1 pound black beans, picked over, rinsed and soaked overnight

7 cups water

2 tablespoons pure-pressed extra virgin olive oil

1 medium chopped onion

2 minced garlic cloves

1 small diced fresh jalapeño pepper; or 1 to 2 tablespoons canned diced green chilies, to taste [wear rubber gloves to prepare fresh jalapeño pepper]

1 green bell pepper, chopped

2 teaspoons ground cumin

2 teaspoons dried oregano

1 teaspoon chili powder

2 bay leaves

½ teaspoon red-pepper flakes

28 ounces canned tomatoes, chopped (reserve liquid)

2 tablespoons chopped fresh cilantro

freshly ground black pepper, to taste

1 tablespoon fresh lime juice

Topping

2 cups grated Monterey Jack cheese

1 cup whole sour cream

Drain black beans after soaking overnight. In a heavy-bottomed soup pot, cover beans with water and bring to a boil. Reduce heat to medium and cook uncovered until beans are tender, about 45 minutes to 1 hour, skimming off any foam that may collect on the surface.

In a large nonstick skillet, heat oil over medium-high heat. When oil is hot, add onion, garlic, jalapeño pepper, bell pepper, cumin, oregano and chili powder. Sauté until vegetables are softened and tender, about 10 minutes.

Add sautéed vegetables, bay leaves, red-pepper flakes, tomatoes and their juice, cilantro and black pepper to cooked beans. Cook over low heat 30 minutes. Add lime juice. Taste, and adjust seasonings. Ladle into bowls and top with grated cheese and a spoonful of sour cream.

Broccoli Cheese Pie

Makes 6 servings • Each serving: 14 grams protein • 2 grams carbohydrate

2 tablespoons unsalted butter

⅔ cup thinly sliced scallions

2½ cups steamed broccoli, cut into bite-size florets, with stalks trimmed and chopped; or 20 ounces packaged frozen broccoli, thawed, drained and chopped

1½ cups whole cottage cheese or whole ricotta cheese

3 beaten eggs

2 ounces crumbled Gorgonzola or any other blue-veined cheese

¼ cup minced fresh parsley

2 tablespoons fresh slivered basil, or 2 teaspoons dried basil

3 tablespoons flour

freshly ground black pepper, to taste

dash cayenne pepper

2 tablespoons grated Parmesan cheese

Preheat oven to 350°. In a large nonstick skillet, melt butter over medium-high heat. When butter is hot and bubbly, reduce heat to medium. Add scallions and sauté until softened, about 3 minutes. In a large bowl, using a fork, blend sautéed scallions, broccoli, cottage cheese or ricotta cheese, eggs, Gorgonzola cheese, parsley, basil, flour, black pepper and cayenne pepper.

Pour filling into a buttered 9-inch baking pan or soufflé dish.* Top with Parmesan cheese and bake until puffed up and golden brown, about 30 to 35 minutes. Broil for 1 minute to brown top. Let cool 5 minutes before slicing.

———————

Or prepare a rice crust (see Rice Crust recipe, page 205). Rice crust only: 3 grams protein • 21 grams carbohydrate

Broiled Skewered Sesame Tofu with Hot Mustard Sauce

Makes 4 servings • Each serving: 27 grams protein • trace carbohydrate

1½ pounds firm tofu, drained, pressed and cut into 1½-inch cubes (for directions, see "All You Need to Know About Tofu," page 10)

2 to 4 tablespoons low-sodium tamari soy sauce, to taste

¼ cup pure-pressed sesame oil

2 tablespoons rice wine vinegar

1 tablespoon dry sherry

1 tablespoon fresh lime juice

1 tablespoon minced scallions

1 tablespoon minced fresh cilantro

1 tablespoon peeled and finely minced fresh ginger

1 minced clove garlic

dash cayenne pepper

1 bell pepper, cut into 1½-inch squares

16 brown or white mushrooms

2 small zucchini, sliced into ¼-inch slices

eight 8-inch bamboo skewers soaked in water 15 minutes to prevent burning

Hot Mustard Sauce

Prepare tofu and set aside. In a large flat container, combine soy sauce, sesame oil, rice wine vinegar, sherry, lime juice, scallions, cilantro, ginger, garlic and cayenne pepper. Add tofu, bell pepper, mushrooms and zucchini. Mix well and marinate, refrigerated and covered, at least 1 hour, or overnight if possible.

Preheat broiler. Thread marinated tofu on skewers, alternating with bell peppers, mushrooms and zucchini. Arrange skewers on a greased rack with a tinfoil-lined baking sheet underneath. Broil until browned, about 7 to 10 minutes on each side. Brush with marinade. Serve with Hot Mustard Sauce.

Hot Mustard Sauce

3 tablespoons dried hot mustard

2 tablespoons water

1 tablespoon low-sodium tamari soy sauce

1 teaspoon fresh lime juice

In a small bowl, using a fork, mix ingredients until well blended.

Broiled Tofu Sandwich

Makes 4 servings • Each serving: 24 grams protein • 46 grams carbohydrate
To reduce carbohydrates, use a low-carbohydrate bread.

∽

*1 pound firm tofu, drained,
pressed, sliced into 4 crosswise
slices and marinated
(for directions, see "All You
Need to Know About Tofu,"
page 10)*

4 slices mozzarella cheese

8 slices whole-grain bread

*mayonnaise (made from pure-
pressed oil)*

mustard

4 slices tomato

4 slices red onion

2 thinly sliced ripe avocados

4 leaves romaine lettuce

Preheat broiler. Arrange marinated tofu slices on a greased rack with a tinfoil-lined baking sheet underneath. Broil until browned, about 5 to 7 minutes per side. Add cheese to top for last minute of broiling.

Toast bread, if desired. Make a sandwich with bread, broiled tofu and cheese, mayonnaise, mustard, tomato, onion, avocado and lettuce.

Cheesy Enchiladas

Makes 8 servings • Each serving: 20 grams protein • 30 grams carbohydrate

3 tablespoons pure-pressed
extra virgin olive oil

1 large diced onion

2 minced garlic cloves

4 ounces canned diced green
chilies

1 teaspoon ground cumin

1 teaspoon dried oregano

freshly ground black pepper,
to taste

2 cups whole cottage cheese

2 tablespoons minced scallions

2 tablespoons minced fresh cilantro

2 cups grated Monterey Jack
cheese

4 cups Enchilada Sauce
(see recipe, page 305), or
store-bought

12 corn tortillas

1 tablespoon minced scallions,
for garnish

1 tablespoon minced fresh
cilantro, for garnish

2 tablespoons chopped black
olives, for garnish

1 cup whole sour cream, for
topping

Preheat oven to 350°. In a large nonstick skillet, heat oil over medium-high heat. When oil is hot, add onion, garlic, chilies, cumin, oregano and black pepper. Sauté until softened, about 5 minutes.

In a large bowl, using a fork, mix sautéed vegetable mixture, cottage cheese, scallions, cilantro and 1 cup Monterey Jack cheese.

In a medium saucepan, heat enchilada sauce until hot and bubbly. Pour 1 cup of sauce into bottom of a 9×13-inch baking dish. Dip tortillas, one at a time, in remaining simmering enchilada sauce about 5 seconds to soften, thoroughly coating both sides. Using tongs, transfer each tortilla to a plate. Spoon about ¼ cup filling on each tortilla, just off center. Roll tortilla around filling and place seam-side down in baking pan. Repeat with remaining tortillas.

Spread remaining sauce over filled tortillas. Top with 1 cup grated cheese. Bake, uncovered, 25 minutes, until hot and bubbly. Sprinkle with scallions, cilantro and black olives. Serve with a spoonful of sour cream.

Cheesy Polenta with Eggplant Tomato Sauce

Makes 6 servings • Each serving: 17 grams protein • 38 grams carbohydrate

4 cups vegetable stock (see recipe, page 100), or low-sodium canned or water

1 cup polenta

½ cup grated mozzarella cheese

1 medium eggplant (peeled, if desired), cut into 1½-inch chunks

¼ cup pure-pressed extra virgin olive oil

freshly ground black pepper, to taste

3 cups Basic Tomato Sauce (see recipe, page 300), or store-bought

1 cup grated mozzarella cheese

½ cup grated Parmesan cheese

2 tablespoons minced fresh parsley

In a large heavy-bottomed saucepan, bring vegetable stock or water to a boil over high heat. Reduce heat to medium. Sprinkle polenta into boiling stock in a steady slow stream, whisking almost constantly until mixture is thickened and smooth, about 20 minutes. Reduce heat to low, stir in ½ cup mozzarella cheese and cook 5 more minutes, stirring. Pour into a 9×13-inch pan and set aside.

Preheat oven to 400°. Toss eggplant with olive oil and black pepper and spread in a single layer on a greased baking sheet. Roast 20 minutes or until tender and evenly browned, turning occasionally. Remove from oven and reduce oven temperature to 350°.

Spread roasted eggplant over polenta, top with tomato sauce and sprinkle with remaining grated mozzarella and Parmesan cheeses. Cover and bake until heated through, about 20 minutes. Uncover to brown top during last 10 minutes of baking. Sprinkle with minced parsley before serving.

Cheesy Quesadillas

Makes 4 servings • Each serving: 27 grams protein • 39 grams carbohydrate
(Nutritional information does not include salsa)

Filling

2 ounces canned diced green
   chilies

1½ cups diced baked tofu, heated
   (for directions, see "All You
   Need to Know About Tofu,"
   page 10)

1 tablespoon pure-pressed
   monounsaturated vegetable oil

¼ cup minced scallions

2 tablespoons minced fresh cilantro

1½ cups grated Monterey Jack
   cheese

8 corn tortillas

Topping

2 thinly sliced ripe avocados

1 cup whole sour cream

½ cup salsa (see Salsas, starting
   on page 296), or store-bought

In a medium bowl, combine filling ingredients.

In a medium nonstick skillet, heat oil over medium heat. When oil is hot, add a tortilla and heat on one side before flipping over.

Spoon ½ cup of filling on half of tortilla, being careful not to over-fill. Fold tortilla in half.

Cook each side about 2 to 3 minutes, until cheese is melted and filling is hot. Add more oil to pan if needed and cook remaining tortillas the same way. Add sliced avocado and sour cream before serving. Serve salsa on the side.

Coconut Cashew Nut Curry

Makes 4 servings • Each serving: 15 grams protein • 39 grams carbohydrate
½ cup brown rice: 3 grams protein • 23 grams carbohydrate

*1½ cups raw cashew nuts, for
topping*

*2 tablespoons pure-pressed
monounsaturated vegetable oil*

1 tablespoon unsalted butter

1 medium chopped onion

2 minced garlic cloves

*1 small diced fresh jalapeño
pepper; or 1 to 2 tablespoons
canned diced green chilies, to
taste* [wear rubber gloves to
prepare fresh jalapeño pepper]

1 red bell pepper, sliced into slivers

*2 large diced red potatoes
(peeled, if desired)*

*1 medium head cauliflower, cut
into florets*

1 teaspoon ground turmeric

1 teaspoon ground cumin

1 teaspoon ground coriander

½ teaspoon ground cardamom

*2 teaspoons peeled and finely
minced fresh ginger*

1 cinnamon stick

dash cayenne pepper

1½ cups coconut milk

*½ cup vegetable stock (see recipe,
page 100), or low-sodium
canned or water*

*1 cup fresh green peas or frozen
and thawed*

*1 to 2 teaspoons fresh lime juice,
to taste*

Put cashews in an ungreased skillet over medium-high heat. Stir nuts or shake pan almost constantly until cashews are evenly browned and toasted. Remove from pan immediately and set aside.

In a large nonstick skillet, heat oil and butter over medium-high heat. When hot, add onion, garlic, jalapeño pepper and bell pepper. Sauté until softened, about 5 minutes. Add potatoes, cauliflower, turmeric, cumin, coriander, cardamom, ginger, cinnamon stick and cayenne pepper. Sauté until spices and vegetables are well blended and coated with oil, stirring constantly, about 2 minutes.

Add coconut milk and vegetable stock or water. Bring to a boil. Reduce heat to low and simmer until potatoes are tender and sauce is thickened, about 15 to 20 minutes.

Stir in peas and lime juice and cook until heated through. Sprinkle with toasted cashews. Serve over steamed brown rice.

Curried Tofu with Vegetables

Makes 4 servings • Each serving: 13 grams protein • 13 grams carbohydrate
½ cup brown rice: 3 grams protein • 23 grams carbohydrate

8 garlic cloves

2-inch piece fresh ginger, peeled and coarsely chopped

1 small chopped fresh jalapeño pepper; or 1 to 2 tablespoons canned diced green chilies, to taste [wear rubber gloves to prepare fresh jalapeño pepper]

¼ cup vegetable stock (see recipe, page 100), or low-sodium canned, or water

3 tablespoons pure-pressed extra virgin olive oil

2 teaspoons ground coriander

2 teaspoons ground cumin

1 teaspoon ground turmeric

dash cayenne pepper

1½ pounds firm tofu, drained, pressed and cut into ½-inch cubes (for directions, see "All You Need to Know About Tofu," page 10)

1 medium head cauliflower, cut into small florets and steamed

2 cups steamed diced carrots

2 cups fresh green peas or frozen and thawed

1 to 2 teaspoons fresh lime juice, to taste

2 tablespoons minced fresh cilantro, for garnish

In a blender, purée garlic, ginger, jalapeño pepper and vegetable stock or water until smooth. Set aside.

In a large nonstick skillet, heat oil over medium-high heat. When oil is hot, add garlic purée and sauté, stirring frequently for 1 minute. Add coriander, cumin, turmeric and cayenne pepper. Cook 2 minutes, stirring constantly. Add tofu cubes and sauté until well-coated with spices and browned, about 10 minutes. Add steamed cauliflower, carrots, peas and lime juice and cook until peas are tender and heated through, about 5 minutes.

Taste, and adjust seasonings. Sprinkle with fresh cilantro. Serve over steamed brown rice.

Egg Foo Yung with Rice Crust

Makes 6 servings • Each serving: 10 grams protein • 21 grams carbohydrate

1 tablespoon raw sesame seeds

2½ cups cooked cold brown rice

2 tablespoons pure-pressed
   sesame oil

1 beaten egg

1 tablespoon flour

2 tablespoons minced scallions

1 tablespoon low-sodium tamari
   soy sauce

Egg Foo Yung Filling (see recipe,
   page 182)

Put sesame seeds in an ungreased skillet over medium-high heat. Stir seeds or shake pan almost constantly until seeds are evenly browned and toasted and begin to pop. Remove from pan immediately and set aside.

Preheat oven to 350°. Lightly oil a 9-inch pie pan.

In a medium bowl, using a fork, combine cold cooked rice, sesame oil, beaten egg, flour, scallions, sesame seeds and soy sauce. Mix well. Gently pat rice mixture into pie pan, pressing against the edges and bottom of pan with the back of a fork. Bake 20 minutes until evenly browned.

Egg Foo Yung Filling

2 tablespoons pure-pressed
   peanut oil

1 minced garlic clove

1 teaspoon peeled and finely
   minced fresh ginger

½ diced red or green bell pepper

1 cup grated carrots

1 cup diced celery stalks

1 cup grated zucchini

1 cup sliced brown or white
   mushrooms

¼ cup minced scallions

1 cup bean sprouts

4 eggs

1 tablespoon pure-pressed sesame
   oil

1 tablespoon low-sodium tamari
   soy sauce

dash cayenne pepper

In a wok or a large nonstick skillet, heat peanut oil over medium-high heat. When oil is hot, add garlic and ginger and stir-fry 30 seconds, stirring often. Add bell pepper, carrots, celery, zucchini, mushrooms, scallions and bean sprouts and stir-fry 4 to 5 minutes. Transfer to a medium bowl, pressing out and draining excess liquid.

In a small bowl, using a fork, beat eggs, sesame oil, soy sauce and cayenne pepper. Pour over vegetable mixture, mix well and pour into baked rice crust. Bake until filling is browned and set, about 30 minutes.

Eggplant Parmigiana

Makes 4 servings • Each serving: 24 grams protein • 21 grams carbohydrate

*1 large eggplant (peeled, if
  desired)*

¼ cup flour

*freshly ground black pepper,
  to taste*

*¼ cup pure-pressed extra virgin
  olive oil*

*2 cups Basic Tomato Sauce
  (see recipe, page 300), or
  store-bought (no sugar added)*

1 teaspoon dried oregano

2 cups grated mozzarella cheese

½ cup grated Parmesan cheese

Preheat oven to 375°. Slice eggplant crosswise into ½-inch slices.
Dredge slices with flour mixed with black pepper.

In a large nonstick skillet, heat 2 tablespoons of oil over medium-
high heat. When oil is hot, add a few eggplant slices and sauté until
softened and browned, about 5 minutes on each side. Repeat with
remaining oil and eggplant slices.

Spread ½ cup of tomato sauce in a 9×13-inch baking dish. Add a
single layer of eggplant slices. Top with ¾ cup of sauce and ½ teaspoon oregano. Sprinkle with 1 cup mozzarella cheese and ¼ cup
Parmesan cheese. Make a second layer with the rest of the eggplant,
tomato sauce, oregano, mozzarella cheese and Parmesan cheese. Bake,
uncovered, until hot and bubbly, about 20 to 25 minutes.

Eggplant Rollatini

Makes 4 servings • Each serving: 36 grams protein • 22 grams carbohydrate

1 egg, beaten

1 pound whole ricotta cheese

1 teaspoon grated lemon zest

1 cup grated mozzarella cheese

½ cup grated Parmesan cheese

2 tablespoons minced fresh parsley

1 teaspoon dried basil

1 teaspoon dried oregano

freshly ground black pepper, to taste

1 large eggplant

¼ cup flour

¼ cup pure-pressed extra virgin olive oil

2 cups Basic Tomato Sauce (see recipe, page 300), or store-bought (no sugar added)

½ cup all-dairy heavy cream

¼ cup grated Parmesan cheese

Preheat oven to 375°. In a large bowl, using a fork, blend beaten egg, ricotta cheese, lemon zest, mozzarella cheese, Parmesan cheese, parsley, basil, oregano and black pepper. Set aside.

Slice the whole, unpeeled eggplant lengthwise into ¼-inch slices. Dredge with flour. In a large nonstick skillet, heat 2 tablespoons oil over medium-high heat. When oil is hot, add a few eggplant slices in a single layer and sauté until softened and browned, about 3 to 5 minutes on each side. Repeat with remaining oil and eggplant slices.

In a medium bowl, using a fork, combine tomato sauce and cream. Pour 1 cup of sauce into a 10-inch glass pie pan or similar-size baking dish. Spoon about 1 to 2 tablespoons filling at top end of each slice of eggplant. Roll eggplant around filling and place seam-side down into baking dish. Repeat with remaining eggplant and filling.

Pour remaining sauce over eggplant. Sprinkle with Parmesan cheese and bake until sauce is hot and bubbly, about 20 to 25 minutes.

Falafel Balls with Tahini Sauce

Makes 4 servings • Each serving: 18 grams protein • 39 grams carbohydrate
2 tablespoons Tahini Sauce: 1 gram protein • 1 gram carbohydrate

1 (15 ounce) can garbanzo
  beans, drained and rinsed

2 minced garlic cloves

½ cup water

½ pound firm tofu, drained,
  pressed and crumbled
  (for directions, see "All You
  Need to Know About Tofu,"
  page 10)

1 cup fresh or dried whole-grain
  bread crumbs

1 tablespoon pure-pressed extra
  virgin olive oil

2 tablespoons minced fresh
  parsley

freshly ground black pepper,
  to taste

dash cayenne pepper

1 teaspoon ground cumin

1 teaspoon ground coriander

½ teaspoon ground turmeric

2 tablespoons flour

2 tablespoons pure-pressed extra
  virgin olive oil

Tahini Sauce (see recipe,
  page 186)

In a food processor, combine garbanzo beans, garlic and water until well blended. Transfer to a large bowl. Add crumbled tofu, bread crumbs, olive oil, parsley, black pepper, cayenne pepper, cumin, coriander and turmeric, and mix well with a fork. Form into 1½-inch balls or small patties. Roll balls or patties in flour.

In a large nonstick skillet, heat oil over medium-high heat. When oil is hot, sauté falafel balls, turning occasionally, until golden brown and heated through. Falafel balls can also be baked in a 375° oven on a lightly oiled baking sheet for about 20 minutes. Turn occasionally to brown evenly.

Serve with Tahini Sauce (see recipe, page 186).

Tahini Sauce

½ cup sesame tahini

½ cup whole plain yogurt

¼ cup fresh lemon juice

2 minced garlic cloves

1 teaspoon ground cumin

freshly ground black pepper,
  to taste

dash cayenne pepper

In a blender or food processor, combine all ingredients and blend until smooth. Taste, and adjust seasonings.

Makes about 1¼ cups.

Feta Cheese and Mushroom Quesadillas

Makes 4 servings • Each serving: 14 grams protein • 26 grams carbohydrate

2 tablespoons pure-pressed extra
  virgin olive oil, or unsalted
  butter

1 medium chopped red onion

1 minced garlic clove

1 diced red or green bell pepper

1 teaspoon ground cumin

1 teaspoon chili powder

1 teaspoon dried oregano

dash cayenne pepper

freshly ground black pepper,
  to taste

3 cups sliced brown or white
  mushrooms

1 cup crumbled feta cheese

2 tablespoons minced fresh
  parsley

2 medium diced ripe tomatoes

4 corn tortillas

2 thinly sliced ripe avocados
  (optional)

In a large nonstick skillet, heat oil or butter over medium-high heat. When hot, add onion, garlic, bell pepper, cumin, chili powder, oregano, cayenne pepper and black pepper. Sauté until vegetables are almost tender, about 5 minutes, stirring often. Add mushrooms and sauté until softened, about 5 minutes. Remove from heat, add feta cheese, parsley and tomatoes, and mix until cheese melts.

Heat tortillas by placing them one at a time over an open flame and turning with tongs until puffed up and softened; *or* layer tortillas between paper towels and microwave on high for 10 to 20 seconds until heated and puffed up.

Mound ¼ of filling on each tortilla. Top with avocado slices.

Greek-Salad-Filled Pita Breads

Makes 4 servings • Each serving: 13 grams protein • 35 grams carbohydrate

4 whole-grain pita breads

8 large romaine leaves

⅔ cup crumbled feta cheese

¼ cup sliced Kalamata olives

2 chopped celery stalks

1 cup marinated artichoke
hearts, drained and coarsely
chopped

1 small diced red onion

1 chopped small tomato

1 diced red bell pepper

2 tablespoons minced fresh
parsley

2 tablespoons minced fresh mint

1 teaspoon dried oregano

1 tablespoon fresh lemon juice

2 tablespoons pure-pressed extra
virgin olive oil

freshly ground black pepper,
to taste

Cut pita breads in half and line with a romaine leaf.

In a large bowl, combine all remaining ingredients and mix well.
Taste, and adjust seasonings. Fill pita breads with Greek salad and
serve immediately.

Indonesian Tofu Saté
with Peanut Sauce

Makes 4 servings • Each serving: 30 grams protein • 4 grams carbohydrate

*1½ pounds firm tofu, drained,
pressed and cut into 1½-inch
pieces (for directions, see
"All You Need to Know About
Tofu," page 10)*

Marinade

*4 tablespoons organic peanut
butter, smooth or chunky
(no honey or sugar added)*

*2 tablespoons low-sodium tamari
soy sauce*

2 tablespoons fresh lime juice

*1 tablespoon peeled and finely
minced fresh ginger*

2 minced garlic cloves

*1 tablespoon chopped fresh
cilantro*

dash cayenne pepper

*eight 8-inch bamboo skewers
soaked in water 15 minutes to
prevent burning*

Prepare tofu and set aside. In a blender or food processor, blend marinade ingredients until smooth. Add 1 to 2 teaspoons hot water if needed to thin marinade. Taste, and adjust seasonings.

Mix tofu with peanut sauce marinade. Place in covered container, and marinate, refrigerated, at least 30 minutes, or overnight if possible, turning occasionally.

Preheat broiler. Thread tofu on skewers. Arrange skewers on a greased rack with a tinfoil-lined baking sheet underneath. Broil, turning occasionally, until evenly browned, about 10 minutes per side. Brush with extra marinade before serving.

Kasha with Broccoli and Mushrooms in Cream Sauce

Makes 6 servings • Each serving: 9 grams protein • 25 grams carbohydrate

1¼ cups kasha

1 beaten egg

2½ cups boiling vegetable stock
(see recipe, page 100), or
low-sodium canned, or water

Broccoli and Mushroom Sauce
(see recipe, page 191)

In a medium saucepan, combine kasha and egg and stir over medium heat until kasha has absorbed all of the egg and grains are separate and dry-looking, about 3 minutes.

Add boiling stock or water. Cover and simmer over low heat until liquid is absorbed, about 10 to 12 minutes. Remove from heat and let stand, covered, 5 minutes before fluffing with a fork. Serve with Broccoli and Mushroom Sauce (see recipe, page 191).

Broccoli and Mushroom Sauce

½ cup diced raw walnuts

3 tablespoons unsalted butter

1 large diced onion

2 minced garlic cloves

1 pound sliced brown or white
mushrooms

1 bunch broccoli, cut into
bite-size florets, with stalks
trimmed and chopped; or
10 ounces packaged frozen
broccoli, thawed, drained
and chopped

2 tablespoons fresh slivered basil,
or 2 teaspoons dried basil

½ teaspoon dried thyme

2 tablespoons minced fresh
parsley

1 tablespoon low-sodium tamari
soy sauce

freshly ground black pepper,
to taste

dash cayenne pepper

1 cup whole sour cream

Put walnuts in an ungreased nonstick skillet over medium-high heat. Stir nuts or shake pan almost constantly until walnuts are evenly browned and toasted. Remove from pan immediately and set aside.

In a large nonstick skillet, melt butter over medium-high heat. When butter is hot and bubbly, add onion and garlic and sauté until softened, about 5 minutes. Add mushrooms and broccoli and sauté until softened and tender, about 8 minutes. Reduce heat to low, add basil, thyme, parsley, tamari soy sauce, black pepper, cayenne pepper and sour cream. Cook 3 minutes, until hot and bubbly. *Do not boil.* Taste, and adjust seasonings. Sprinkle with diced walnuts. Serve over kasha.

Note: Broccoli and Mushroom Sauce may also be used as a topping for baked potatoes.

Meatless Moussaka

Makes 8 servings • Each serving: 17 grams protein • 11 grams carbohydrate

*3 large eggplants (peeled,
if desired)*

*½ cup pure-pressed extra virgin
olive oil*

*⅔ cup Parmesan cheese (to be
reserved for later use)*

*4 cups Tomato Sauce (see recipe,
below),* or *store-bought
(no sugar added)*

*Ricotta Topping (see recipe,
page 193)*

Preheat broiler. Slice eggplant into ½-inch crosswise slices. Brush both sides with oil and arrange on a greased rack with a tinfoil-lined baking sheet underneath. Broil 3 to 5 minutes per side until evenly browned and tender. Set aside. Prepare tomato sauce and filling and set aside until ready to assemble.

Tomato Sauce

*3 tablespoons pure-pressed extra
virgin olive oil*

1 cup minced onion

2 minced garlic cloves

*4 cups tomatoes, chopped
(reserve liquid)*

1 tablespoon tomato paste

¾ teaspoon ground cinnamon

½ teaspoon dried oregano

In a medium saucepan, heat oil over medium-high heat. When oil is hot, add onion and garlic and sauté until softened, about 5 minutes. Add tomatoes and their liquid, tomato paste, cinnamon and oregano. Bring to a boil, reduce heat to low and simmer until sauce is thickened, about 20 minutes. Begin preparing Ricotta Topping (see recipe, page 193).

Ricotta Topping

¼ cup unsalted butter

¼ cup flour

¾ cup all-dairy heavy cream

¾ cup water

¼ teaspoon ground nutmeg

¼ teaspoon white pepper

4 beaten eggs

2 cups whole ricotta cheese

Preheat oven to 350°. In a large nonstick skillet, melt butter over medium-high heat. When butter is hot and bubbly, reduce heat to low, sprinkle in flour and cook over low heat, stirring constantly, 3 minutes.

In a small bowl, using a fork, combine cream and water. Add liquid to flour mixture in a steady stream, whisking until smooth. Add nutmeg and white pepper. Simmer sauce over low heat 15 minutes or until thickened, stirring occasionally. *Do not boil.* Remove from heat and let cool 10 minutes.

In a large bowl, using a fork, combine beaten eggs and ricotta cheese. Add sauce in a steady stream, whisking until filling is smooth and thoroughly blended.

Spread ½ of tomato sauce in bottom of 10×15-inch baking dish. Top with ½ of the eggplant slices. Sprinkle with ⅓ cup Parmesan cheese. Add remaining tomato sauce and eggplant slices, and pour ricotta topping over eggplant. Sprinkle with ⅓ cup Parmesan cheese and bake about 50 minutes, until top is set and lightly browned. Let stand 20 minutes before serving.

Moroccan Stew with Couscous

Makes 6 servings • Each serving: 5 grams protein • 16 grams carbohydrate
(Nutritional information does not include couscous)

3 tablespoons pure-pressed extra virgin olive oil

1 cup chopped red onion

1 chopped red bell pepper

1 minced garlic clove

2 teaspoons ground cumin

1 teaspoon cinnamon

1 teaspoon ground ginger

2 teaspoons paprika

1 teaspoon chili powder

1 large eggplant (peeled, if desired) and cubed into ½-inch pieces

1 medium head cauliflower, cut into bite-size florets

3 diced medium zucchini

28 ounces canned tomatoes, chopped (reserve liquid)

15 ounces canned rinsed and drained garbanzo beans

¼ cup minced fresh parsley

¼ cup minced fresh cilantro

1 to 2 tablespoons fresh lemon juice, to taste

freshly ground black pepper, to taste

Couscous (see recipe, page 195)

In a large heavy-bottomed soup pot, heat oil over medium-high heat. When oil is hot, add onion, bell pepper and garlic and sauté until softened, about 5 minutes. Add cumin, cinnamon, ginger, paprika, chili powder and eggplant. Sauté until vegetables are well-coated with oil and spices, about 7 minutes.

Add cauliflower, zucchini, tomatoes and their liquid. Bring to a boil. Cover, reduce heat to low and simmer until all vegetables are tender, about 20 minutes. Add garbanzo beans, parsley, cilantro, lemon juice and black pepper. Taste, and adjust seasonings. Serve over Couscous (see recipe, page 195).

Couscous

Makes 2¹/₂ cups • Each ¹/₃ cup serving: 2 grams protein • 14 grams carbohydrate

*1 cup boiling vegetable stock
(see recipe, page 100), or
low-sodium canned, or water*

1 tablespoon unsalted butter
1 cup couscous

In a medium saucepan, bring stock and butter to a boil over high heat. Put dry couscous in another pot. Pour hot stock or water over couscous. Stir once, cover with a tight-fitting lid and remove from heat. Let stand 10 minutes until all liquid is absorbed. Fluff with a fork. Serve immediately.

Mushroom Quiche with Potato Crust

Makes 6 servings • Each serving: 16 grams protein • 8 grams carbohydrate

2 cups packed, grated raw russet
potato (peeled, if desired)

¼ cup grated onion

1 beaten egg

freshly ground black pepper,
to taste

Filling

2 tablespoons unsalted butter

1 medium diced onion, or 1 cup
well-washed, finely chopped
leeks

2 cups sliced brown or white
mushrooms

4 eggs

1 cup all-dairy heavy cream

½ cup water

dash cayenne pepper

dash nutmeg

1½ cups grated Gruyère or
Monterey Jack cheese

Preheat oven to 375°. Grate potatoes and squeeze out excess liquid with paper towels. In a large bowl, using a fork, combine potatoes, grated onion, egg and black pepper. Pat mixture into a well-greased 10-inch pie pan. Bake 35 minutes, until evenly browned.

Prepare quiche filling. In a large skillet, melt butter over medium-high heat. When butter is hot and bubbly, add onion or leeks and sauté until softened, about 5 minutes. Add mushrooms and sauté until tender, about 5 to 7 minutes. Remove from heat, drain off any excess liquid and set aside.

In a large bowl, using a fork, beat eggs. Add cream, water, cayenne pepper and nutmeg, mixing well. Pour mushroom and onion mixture into pie pan. Cover with grated cheese. Pour egg mixture carefully over top of cheese, being careful not to overfill pan. (Extra custard may be baked separately in a greased ramekin.)

Bake 20 to 30 minutes, or until filling is set. When done, a knife inserted into center will come out clean. Cool 10 minutes before serving.

Mushroom Tofu Burger

Makes 4 servings • Each serving: 44 grams protein • 48 grams carbohydrate
Served without bun: 40 grams protein • 33 grams carbohydrate

3 tablespoons raw sesame seeds

2 tablespoons pure-pressed
extra virgin olive oil

1 minced garlic clove

½ cup diced onion

½ pound chopped brown or
white mushrooms

1 pound firm tofu, drained,
marinated and crumbled
(for directions, see "All You
Need to Know About Tofu,"
page 10)

½ cup cooked brown rice

½ cup sesame tahini

2 whole-grain buns

8 tomato slices

4 lettuce leaves

½ cup grated carrot

½ cup fresh or dried whole-grain
bread crumbs

½ cup minced scallions

¼ cup minced fresh parsley

1 cup grated mozzarella cheese

1 beaten egg

1 tablespoon low-sodium tamari
soy sauce

freshly ground black pepper,
to taste

dash cayenne pepper

2 tablespoons pure-pressed
extra virgin olive oil

2 sliced ripe avocados

Aioli (Garlic Mayonnaise)
(see recipe, page 290)

Put sesame seeds in an ungreased skillet over medium-high heat. Stir seeds or shake pan almost constantly until seeds are evenly browned and toasted and begin to pop. Remove from pan immediately and set aside.

In a large nonstick skillet, heat 2 tablespoons oil over medium-high heat. When oil is hot, add garlic and onion and sauté until softened, about 3 minutes. Add mushrooms and sauté 3 to 5 minutes. Drain and transfer to a large bowl. Add tofu, rice, sesame tahini, carrot, bread crumbs, scallions, parsley, sesame seeds, mozzarella cheese, egg, tamari soy sauce, black pepper and cayenne pepper. Mix well with a fork.

Shape into 4 large patties. In a large nonstick skillet, heat oil over medium-high heat. When oil is hot, add tofu burgers and cook until browned, about 5 minutes on each side. Serve open-faced on half a whole-grain bun with tomato, lettuce, avocado and Garlic Mayonnaise.

Mushroom Zucchini Quiche
with Rice Crust

Makes 6 servings • Each serving: 14 grams protein • 22 grams carbohydrate

2½ cups cooked brown rice

2 tablespoons melted unsalted
   butter

1 beaten egg

1 tablespoon flour

1 tablespoon minced fresh parsley

2 tablespoons minced scallions

freshly ground black pepper,
   to taste

Mushroom Zucchini Quiche
   Filling (see recipe, page 199)

Preheat oven to 350°. Lightly butter a 9-inch pie pan.

In a medium bowl, using a fork, combine cooked rice with melted butter, egg, flour, parsley, scallions and black pepper. Mix well. Gently pat into pie pan, pressing against the edges and bottom of pan with the back of a fork. Bake 20 minutes, until evenly browned.

Mushroom Zucchini Quiche Filling

2 tablespoons unsalted butter

1 small diced red onion

1 pound thinly sliced zucchini

2 cups sliced brown or white
  mushrooms

1 cup whole cottage cheese or
  whole ricotta cheese

3 eggs

2 tablespoons all-dairy heavy
  cream

2 tablespoons grated Parmesan
  cheese

2 tablespoons slivered fresh basil,
  or 1 teaspoon dried basil

freshly ground black pepper,
  to taste

In a large nonstick skillet, melt butter over medium-high heat. When butter is hot and bubbly, add onion and sauté until softened, about 3 minutes. Add zucchini and mushrooms and sauté until tender, about 7 minutes. Drain well and set aside.

In a medium bowl, combine cottage cheese or ricotta cheese, eggs, cream, Parmesan cheese, basil and black pepper. Mix well, stirring with a fork. Add sautéed vegetables and pour into prepared rice crust. Bake until filling is browned and set, about 30 minutes.

Mushrooms, Snow Peas and Tofu Stir-Fry

Makes 4 servings • Each serving: 33 grams protein • 13 grams carbohydrate
½ cup Basic Steamed Brown Rice: 3 grams protein • 23 grams carbohydrate

1 cup raw cashew nuts, for topping

2 tablespoons pure-pressed peanut oil

1½ pounds firm tofu, drained, pressed and cut into ½-inch cubes (for directions, see "All You Need to Know About Tofu," page 10)

2 tablespoons low-sodium tamari soy sauce

1 tablespoon pure-pressed peanut oil

1 medium red onion, halved lengthwise and sliced in thin slivers

2 cups sliced brown or white mushrooms

2 minced garlic cloves

1 tablespoon peeled and finely minced fresh ginger

½ pound snow peas, strings removed

1 tablespoon pure-pressed sesame oil

Put cashews in an ungreased skillet over medium-high heat. Stir nuts or shake pan almost constantly until cashews are evenly browned and toasted. Remove from pan immediately and set aside.

In a wok or large nonstick skillet, heat 2 tablespoons peanut oil over high heat. When oil is hot, add tofu cubes and soy sauce and stir-fry until golden brown about 10 minutes, stirring often. Remove from wok or skillet and set aside. Heat remaining 1 tablespoon peanut oil in wok or skillet over high heat. Add onion and stir-fry 2 minutes. Add mushrooms, garlic and ginger and stir-fry 3 minutes. Add snow peas and cooked tofu and cook until snow peas turn bright green, about 1 minute. Drizzle with sesame oil and sprinkle with toasted cashew nuts. Serve over Basic Steamed Brown Rice (see recipe, page 242).

Mushrooms and Sun-Dried Tomato Pesto Polenta

Makes 4 servings • Each serving: 19 grams protein • 53 grams carbohydrate

4 cups vegetable stock (see recipe,
   page 100), or low-sodium
   canned, or water

1 cup polenta

2 tablespoons unsalted butter

2 cups sliced brown or white
   mushrooms

½ cup Sun-Dried Tomato Pesto
   (see recipe, page 295), or
   store-bought

1 cup crumbled feta cheese

1 tablespoon fresh slivered basil,
   or 1 teaspoon dried basil

freshly ground black pepper,
   to taste

In a large saucepan, bring vegetable stock or water to a boil over high heat. Reduce heat to low and sprinkle in polenta in a slow steady stream, stirring constantly. Continue stirring until mixture is thickened and smooth, about 15 to 20 minutes. Set aside.

In a medium nonstick skillet, melt butter over medium heat. When butter is hot and bubbly, add mushrooms and sauté until softened and liquid is absorbed, about 5 to 7 minutes. Add sun-dried pesto, crumbled feta cheese and basil. Season to taste with black pepper. Taste, and adjust seasonings. Cook until heated through. Pour polenta into a serving dish and serve immediately.

Ricotta-Stuffed Bell Peppers

Makes 6 servings • Each serving: 24 grams protein • 11 grams carbohydrate

*4 green or red bell peppers, cut in
  half lengthwise*

1½ pounds whole ricotta cheese

2 eggs

½ cup chopped Kalamata olives

1 cup chopped raw walnuts

½ cup minced fresh parsley

*2 tablespoons slivered fresh basil,
  or 2 teaspoons dried basil*

1 tablespoon grated lemon zest

*freshly ground black pepper,
  to taste*

⅔ cup grated Parmesan cheese

Preheat oven to 350°. Cut bell peppers in half and remove seeds. In a large skillet, bring 2 cups of water to a boil. Add bell peppers, reduce heat to low and simmer until just tender, about 5 minutes. Remove from pan, drain and set aside to cool.

In a medium bowl, combine ricotta cheese, eggs, olives, walnuts, parsley, basil, lemon zest and black pepper. Mix well with a fork. Mound into pepper halves. Sprinkle with Parmesan cheese. Place in an ovenproof baking dish and add water to ¼-inch depth in dish to prevent burning. Bake until heated through, about 20 to 30 minutes. Place under broiler briefly to brown.

Risotto with Mushrooms, Sun-Dried Tomatoes and Gorgonzola Cheese

Makes 8 servings • Each serving: 19 grams protein • 35 grams carbohydrate

1 cup raw pine nuts, for garnish

3 tablespoons pure-pressed extra virgin olive oil, or oil from sun-dried tomatoes

2 minced garlic cloves

1 small diced onion

½ pound thinly sliced brown or white mushrooms

½ cup sun-dried tomatoes, drained and slivered

1½ cups long-grain brown rice, rinsed and drained

5 cups vegetable stock (see recipe, page 100), or low-sodium canned

¼ cup slivered fresh basil, or 2 teaspoons dried basil

1 cup crumbled Gorgonzola cheese

2 teaspoons grated lemon zest

¼ cup all-dairy heavy cream

freshly ground black pepper, to taste

Put pine nuts in an ungreased skillet over medium-high heat. Stir nuts or shake pan almost constantly until pine nuts are evenly browned and toasted. Remove from pan immediately and set aside.

In a large saucepan, heat oil over medium-high heat. When oil is hot, add garlic, onion and mushrooms and sauté until softened, about 5 minutes. Add sun-dried tomatoes and long-grain brown rice and stir gently to thoroughly coat grains of rice with oil.

In another saucepan, bring stock to a boil and reduce heat to low. Ladle 1 cup of simmering stock into rice and stir well. Cook over medium heat, uncovered, stirring constantly until all liquid is absorbed. Add another cup of hot stock and stir constantly until all liquid is absorbed. Continue adding one cup at a time, until all of stock has been absorbed and rice is tender. (Adding stock, cup by cup, will take about 20 to 30 minutes.)

After all stock has been added and rice is cooked to your liking, add basil, Gorgonzola cheese, lemon zest, cream and black pepper. Taste, and adjust seasonings. Sprinkle with pine nuts.

Spinach and Artichoke Gratin with Kalamata Olives

Makes 4 servings • Each serving: 16 grams protein • 24 grams carbohydrate

2 bunches spinach equal to about 2 cups cooked spinach, well drained and chopped; or 16 ounces packaged frozen spinach, thawed, drained and chopped

2 tablespoons unsalted butter

1 small diced red onion

1 minced garlic clove

1 cup marinated artichoke hearts, drained and chopped

¼ cup diced Kalamata olives

1 teaspoon grated lemon zest

1 tablespoon fresh lemon juice

2 tablespoons slivered fresh basil, or 2 teaspoons dried basil

1 teaspoon dried oregano

freshly ground black pepper, to taste

1½ cups cooked brown rice

1 cup crumbled feta cheese

2 tablespoons grated Parmesan cheese, for topping

Wash spinach well, removing stems. With water still clinging to leaves, place in a medium saucepan with a tight-fitting lid. Turn heat to medium-high and steam until leaves are wilted, about 2 to 3 minutes. Drain in a colander, pressing out all liquid with the back of a wooden spoon. Chop coarsely and set aside.

Preheat oven to 350°. In a large nonstick skillet, melt butter over medium-high heat. When butter is hot and bubbly, add onion and garlic and sauté until softened, about 3 minutes.

Stir in spinach, chopped artichoke hearts, olives, lemon zest, lemon juice, basil, oregano and black pepper. Mix well. Stir in cooked brown rice and feta cheese. Pour mixture into a greased 2-quart casserole. Top with Parmesan cheese and bake about 30 minutes until browned and heated through.

Spinach and Feta Cheese with Rice Crust

Makes 6 servings • Each serving: 16 grams protein • 23 grams carbohydrate

Rice Crust

2½ cups cooked brown rice

*2 tablespoons melted unsalted
  butter*

1 egg, beaten

1 tablespoon flour

1 tablespoon minced fresh parsley

*freshly ground black pepper,
  to taste*

*Spinach and Feta Cheese Filling
  (see recipe, page 206)*

Preheat oven to 350°. Lightly butter a 9-inch pie pan.

In a medium bowl, using a fork, combine cooked rice with melted butter, egg, flour, parsley and black pepper. Mix well. Gently pat into pie pan, pressing against edges and bottom of pan with the back of a fork. Bake 20 minutes, until evenly browned.

Spinach and Feta Cheese Filling

2 bunches spinach equal to about
  2 cups cooked spinach, well
  drained and chopped; or
  16 ounces packaged frozen
  spinach, thawed, drained
  and chopped

1 tablespoon pure-pressed extra
  virgin olive oil

1 cup diced scallions

1 minced garlic clove

¼ cup minced fresh parsley

1 teaspoon dill

1 teaspoon dried oregano

4 beaten eggs

1 cup crumbled feta cheese

1 tablespoon flour

1 cup all-dairy heavy cream

freshly ground black pepper,
  to taste

dash cayenne pepper

Wash spinach well, removing stems. With water still clinging to leaves, place in a medium saucepan with a tight-fitting lid. Turn heat to medium-high and steam until leaves are wilted, about 2 to 3 minutes. Drain in a colander, pressing out all liquid with the back of a wooden spoon. Chop coarsely and set aside.

In a large nonstick skillet, heat oil over medium-high heat. When oil is hot, add scallions and garlic and sauté until softened, about 3 minutes. In a medium bowl, combine spinach, scallions, garlic, parsley, dill, oregano, eggs, feta cheese, flour, cream, black pepper and cayenne pepper. Mix well. Pour into prepared rice crust. Bake until filling is browned and set, about 30 minutes.

Szechwan Tofu with Green Beans, Mushrooms and Peanuts

Makes 6 servings • Each serving: 24 grams protein • 4 grams carbohydrate
½ cup Basic Steamed Brown Rice: 3 grams protein • 23 grams carbohydrate

1 ounce dried shitake mushrooms

1 cup hot water

3 tablespoons pure-pressed peanut oil

1½ pounds firm tofu, drained, pressed and cut into ½-inch cubes (for directions, see "All You Need to Know About Tofu," page 10)

2 tablespoons pure-pressed peanut oil

2 minced garlic cloves

1 tablespoon peeled and finely minced fresh ginger

6 scallions cut into 1-inch-long thin slivers

1 small diced fresh jalapeño pepper; or 1 to 2 tablespoons canned diced green chilies, to taste [wear rubber gloves to prepare fresh jalapeño pepper]

1 pound green beans, ends trimmed, sliced diagonally into 2-inch pieces and steamed until tender

1 jicama, peeled and cut into 1-inch-length slivers; or 6 ounces canned sliced water chestnuts, rinsed and drained

2 tablespoons low-sodium tamari soy sauce

2 tablespoons dry sherry

2 tablespoons fresh lime juice

¼ teaspoon red-pepper flakes

2 tablespoons pure-pressed sesame oil

1 cup dry-roasted peanuts

Soak mushrooms in hot water 15 minutes. Remove from water and slice into thin slivers, discarding hard nubs at base of stems. Set aside. (Strain liquid that the mushrooms have been soaking in through a fine-meshed sieve lined with a paper towel, and save for a future soup stock.)

In a wok or a large nonstick skillet, heat 3 tablespoons peanut oil over high heat. When oil is hot, add tofu and stir-fry until browned, turning occasionally, about 10 minutes. Remove from pan and set aside. Repeat in batches, if necessary.

Heat remaining oil over high heat. When oil is hot, add garlic, ginger, scallions and jalapeño pepper. Stir-fry 2 minutes. Add green beans, reserved slivered mushrooms and jicama or water chestnuts. Stir-fry 3 minutes.

Add soy sauce, sherry, lime juice, red-pepper flakes and tofu cubes. Stir-fry until heated through. Drizzle with sesame oil and toss with peanuts. Taste, and adjust seasonings. Serve over Basic Steamed Brown Rice (see recipe, page 242).

Tamale Pie

Makes 8 servings • Each serving: 15 grams protein • 16 grams carbohydrate

3 tablespoons pure-pressed monounsaturated vegetable oil

1 large diced onion

3 minced garlic cloves

1 large diced green bell pepper

1 pound firm tofu, drained, pressed and diced into ¼-inch cubes (for directions, see "All You Need to Know About Tofu," page 10)

1 tablespoon chili powder

1 teaspoon ground cumin

1 teaspoon dried oregano

freshly ground black pepper, to taste

dash cayenne pepper

28 ounces canned crushed tomatoes

13¾ ounces canned kidney beans, drained and rinsed

1 cup fresh corn kernels or frozen and thawed

2 tablespoons minced fresh cilantro

Crust

1½ cups cornmeal

2 teaspoons baking powder

3 tablespoons melted unsalted butter

½ cup all-dairy heavy cream

½ cup water

1 beaten egg

1 cup grated Monterey Jack cheese

Preheat oven to 350°. In a large nonstick skillet, heat oil over medium-high heat. When oil is hot, add onion, garlic, bell pepper, tofu, chili powder, cumin, oregano, black pepper and cayenne pepper and sauté until tofu is browned, about 10 minutes, stirring occasionally. Add tomatoes and their liquid and bring to a boil. Reduce heat to low. Add kidney beans, corn and cilantro. Simmer 5 minutes. Transfer mixture to a lightly greased 2½-quart baking casserole.

In a medium bowl, using a fork, combine cornmeal and baking powder. Mix well. Add butter, cream, water and egg, and stir mixture just until combined. Add grated cheese and mix well. Pour over bean mixture, spreading smoothly over the top. Bake 45 minutes until golden brown.

Tandoori-Style Tofu

Makes 6 servings • Each serving: 25 grams protein • 2 grams carbohydrate
½ cup Indian Rice: 5 grams protein • 26 grams carbohydrate

2 pounds firm tofu, drained,
pressed and sliced into
1 x 3-inch sticks (for directions,
see "All You Need to Know
About Tofu," page 10)

1 cup whole plain yogurt

1 tablespoon peeled and finely
minced fresh ginger

2 minced garlic cloves

1 tablespoon paprika

1 teaspoon ground coriander

1 teaspoon ground cumin

½ teaspoon ground cardamom

¼ teaspoon freshly ground black
pepper

¼ teaspoon cayenne pepper

2 tablespoons minced cilantro

Prepare tofu and set aside. In a large bowl, using a fork, combine yogurt, ginger, garlic, paprika, coriander, cumin, cardamom, black pepper and cayenne pepper. Mix well. Dip tofu sticks into marinade, thoroughly coating on all sides. Marinate at least 30 minutes or overnight, if possible, covered and refrigerated, turning occasionally.

Preheat broiler. Arrange tofu sticks on a greased rack with a tinfoil-lined baking sheet underneath. Broil 8 to 10 minutes on each side until browned, using tongs to turn. Sprinkle with minced cilantro before serving. Serve with Indian Rice (see recipe, page 247).

Tempeh and Cheese Quesadillas

Makes 4 servings • Each serving: 44 grams protein • 35 grams carbohydrate
(Nutritional information does not include salsa)

Tempeh—an Indonesian staple—is another source of complete protein and is high in iron and vitamin B_{12}. It is made by combining cooked soybeans with a mold fungi culture and incubating 24 hours to ferment. The result is a firm, flattened cake with a meaty flavor and chewy texture. Tempeh can be found in most health food stores. It freezes very well.

3 tablespoons pure-pressed
   peanut oil

1 medium chopped onion

1 minced garlic clove

1 diced red or green bell pepper

1 pound tempeh, cubed into
   ½-inch pieces

1 teaspoon ground cumin

1 teaspoon dried oregano

½ cup diced tomatoes

1 tablespoon low-sodium tamari
   soy sauce

2 teaspoons Dijon mustard

freshly ground black pepper,
   to taste

dash hot-pepper sauce

2 tablespoons pure-pressed
   peanut oil, or unsalted butter

4 corn tortillas

Topping

2 cups grated Monterey Jack
   cheese

2 thinly sliced ripe avocados

1 cup whole sour cream

½ cup salsa (see Salsas, starting
   on page 296), or store-bought

In a large nonstick skillet, heat oil over medium-high heat. When oil is hot, add onion, garlic and bell pepper and sauté until softened, about 5 minutes. Add tempeh, cumin and oregano and sauté until lightly browned. Add tomatoes, soy sauce, mustard, black pepper and hot-pepper sauce. Mix well. Taste, and adjust seasonings.

Heat tortillas by placing them one at a time over an open flame and turning with tongs until puffed up and softened; or layer tortillas between paper towels and microwave on high for 10 to 20 seconds until heated and puffed up.

Mound ¼ of tempeh filling on each tortilla. Top with grated cheese and place briefly under broiler to melt cheese. Add sliced avocados and sour cream before serving. Serve salsa on the side.

Tempeh Stir-Fried with Zucchini and Red Bell Pepper

Makes 4 servings • Each serving: 25 grams protein • 9 grams carbohydrate
½ cup Basic Steamed Brown Rice: 3 grams protein • 23 grams carbohydrate

2 tablespoons pure-pressed
  peanut oil

3 minced garlic cloves

1 tablespoon peeled and finely
  minced fresh ginger

½ teaspoon red-pepper flakes

4 medium zucchini, cut into
  ¼-inch half circles

2 slivered red bell peppers

1 pound tempeh, cut into
  ½-inch cubes

2 tablespoons low-sodium tamari
  soy sauce

2 tablespoons dry sherry

2 tablespoons pure-pressed
  sesame oil

1 tablespoon fresh lime juice

2 tablespoons minced scallions

2 tablespoons minced fresh
  cilantro

In a wok or a large nonstick skillet, heat peanut oil over medium-high heat. When oil is hot, add garlic and ginger and cook for 30 seconds, stirring constantly. Add red-pepper flakes, zucchini, red bell pepper and tempeh and stir-fry about 7 minutes, until vegetables are tender.

Combine soy sauce, sherry, sesame oil, lime juice, scallions and cilantro. Pour over tempeh and vegetables and cook, stirring, until heated through. Taste, and adjust seasonings. Serve over Basic Steamed Brown Rice (see recipe, page 242).

Tempeh Tacos

Makes 4 servings • Each serving: 30 grams protein • 34 grams carbohydrate
(Nutritional information does not include salsa)

∼

3 tablespoons pure-pressed
  peanut oil

1 large diced onion

2 minced garlic cloves

4 ounces canned diced chilies

2 teaspoons ground cumin

2 teaspoons dried oregano

2 teaspoons chili powder

1 pound diced tempeh

freshly ground black pepper,
  to taste

4 corn tortillas

Topping

2 diced tomatoes

2 cups shredded green cabbage

2 sliced ripe avocados

1 cup whole sour cream

2 tablespoons chopped fresh
  cilantro

1 cup Mango Salsa (see recipe,
  page 297)

In a large nonstick skillet, heat peanut oil over medium-high heat. When oil is hot, add onion, garlic, chilies, cumin, oregano and chili powder. Sauté until onion is softened, about 5 minutes. Add diced tempeh and cook until lightly browned, about 5 minutes. Season to taste with black pepper.

Heat tortillas by placing them one at a time over an open flame and turning with tongs until puffed up and softened; *or* layer tortillas between paper towels and microwave on high for 10 to 20 seconds until heated and puffed up.

Spoon ¼ of tempeh mixture onto each tortilla and fold into tacos. Top with tomatoes, cabbage, avocados, sour cream, cilantro and salsa.

Tempeh with Eggplant, Zucchini and Tomato

Makes 4 servings • Each serving: 26 grams protein • 9 grams carbohydrate
½ cup Basic Steamed Brown Rice: 3 grams protein • 23 grams carbohydrate

¼ cup pure-pressed extra virgin olive oil

3 minced garlic cloves

1 medium diced onion

1 large diced green or red bell pepper

1 large eggplant (peeled, if desired) cubed into ½-inch pieces

1 pound tempeh, cut into ½-inch cubes

2 medium diced zucchini

2 cups chopped medium tomatoes

2 tablespoons dry red wine

1 teaspoon dried oregano

1 teaspoon dried basil

½ teaspoon dried marjoram

¼ cup minced fresh parsley

½ teaspoon red-pepper flakes

freshly ground black pepper, to taste

In a large nonstick skillet, heat oil over medium-high heat. When oil is hot, add garlic, onion, bell pepper, eggplant and tempeh and cook until softened, about 10 minutes, stirring occasionally. Add remaining ingredients. Bring to a boil, reduce heat to low and simmer 15 to 20 minutes, until vegetables are tender and sauce is thickened, stirring occasionally. Taste, and adjust seasonings. Serve over Basic Steamed Brown Rice (see recipe, page 242).

Thai-Style Tofu

Makes 4 servings • Each serving: 51 grams protein • 16 grams carbohydrate

*2 pounds firm tofu, drained,
pressed and cut into 1½-inch
cubes (for directions, see
"All You Need to Know About
Tofu," page 10)*

Thai Marinade

*1 cup chunky organic peanut
butter (no honey or sugar
added)*

1½ cups coconut milk

*¼ cup vegetable stock (see recipe,
page 100), or low-sodium
canned*

*2 tablespoons low-sodium tamari
soy sauce*

¼ cup fresh lime juice

2 minced garlic cloves

*1 tablespoon peeled and finely
minced fresh ginger*

2 tablespoons chopped scallions

*2 tablespoons chopped fresh
cilantro*

1 tablespoon chopped fresh mint

1 tablespoon slivered fresh basil

*freshly ground black pepper,
to taste*

dash cayenne pepper

*twelve 8-inch wooden skewers,
soaked in water 15 minutes to
prevent burning*

Prepare tofu and set aside. In a large bowl, using a fork, combine marinade ingredients. Mix well. Taste, and adjust seasonings. Thoroughly coat tofu cubes with marinade and marinate, covered and refrigerated, 1 hour or overnight, if possible, turning occasionally.

Prepare barbecue or preheat broiler. Drain and thread tofu onto skewers. Grill over hot coals; *or* broil on a greased rack with a tinfoil-lined baking sheet underneath, turning and basting occasionally, until browned on all sides, about 7 to 10 minutes.

Tofu Enchiladas Suizas

Makes 8 servings • Each serving: 24 grams protein • 29 grams carbohydrate
(Nutritional information does not include salsa)

Salsa Verde

*1 pound tomatillos, husked and
  quartered*

2 chopped garlic cloves

½ small chopped red onion

*1 small chopped fresh jalapeño
  pepper;* or *1 to 2 tablespoons
  canned diced green chilies, to
  taste* [wear rubber gloves to
  prepare fresh jalapeño pepper]

*freshly ground black pepper,
  to taste*

*1¾ cups vegetable stock
  (see recipe, page 100),* or
  low-sodium canned, or *water*

1 cup whole sour cream

*(Ingredient list continues on
  next page)*

Preheat oven to 400°. In a medium saucepan, bring tomatillos, garlic, onion, jalapeño pepper, black pepper and vegetable stock or water
to a boil over medium-high heat. Reduce heat to low and simmer 20
minutes, until onion and tomatillos are softened. In a blender, purée
sauce mixture with sour cream and blend until smooth. Taste, and
adjust seasonings. Pour sauce back into saucepan, reduce heat to low
and simmer while you prepare filling, stirring occasionally. *Do not
boil.* Spoon about ¾ cup of Salsa Verde into a greased 9 × 13-inch
baking pan and set aside.

Enchiladas

1 pound firm tofu, drained,
pressed and crumbled
(for directions, see "All You
Need to Know About Tofu,"
page 10)

1 cup whole cottage cheese

½ cup chopped fresh cilantro

½ cup chopped scallions

4 ounces canned diced green
chilies

½ cup Salsa Verde

½ cup grated Monterey Jack
cheese

freshly ground black pepper,
to taste

cayenne pepper, to taste

12 corn tortillas

1 cup grated Monterey Jack
cheese, for topping

2 tablespoons chopped fresh
cilantro, for garnish

2 tablespoons minced scallions,
for garnish

2 thinly sliced ripe avocados,
for garnish

In a medium bowl, using a fork, combine crumbled tofu, cottage cheese, cilantro, scallions, diced chilies, ½ cup salsa verde, Monterey Jack cheese, black pepper and cayenne pepper. Mix well.

Dip one tortilla at a time into remaining simmering sauce. Soften in sauce about 5 seconds. Using tongs, transfer softened tortilla onto a plate. Spoon ¼ cup of filling in center of each tortilla. Roll tortilla around filling and place seam-side down in baking pan. Repeat with remaining tortillas and filling.

Pour remaining sauce over filled tortillas. Sprinkle with extra 1 cup grated cheese. Bake until enchiladas are hot and cheese is melted, about 25 minutes. Garnish with chopped cilantro, scallions and sliced avocado.

Tofu "Meatballs"

Makes about 18 balls. Each 3-ball serving: 17 grams protein • 17 grams carbohydrate
½ cup Basic Steamed Brown Rice: 3 grams protein • 23 grams carbohydrate

2 tablespoons pure-pressed extra virgin olive oil

1 medium diced onion

2 minced garlic cloves

1 pound firm tofu, drained, pressed and crumbled (for directions, see "All You Need to Know About Tofu," page 10)

¾ cup fresh or dried whole-grain bread crumbs

2 tablespoons organic peanut butter (no honey or sugar added)

3 tablespoons low-sodium tamari soy sauce

2 tablespoons grated Parmesan cheese

½ cup grated carrot

½ cup grated zucchini

2 tablespoons minced fresh parsley

1 teaspoon dried oregano

freshly ground black pepper, to taste

3 tablespoons pure-pressed extra virgin olive oil

4 cups Basic Tomato Sauce (see recipe, page 300), or store-bought

In a medium nonstick skillet, heat oil over medium-high heat. When oil is hot, add onion and garlic and sauté until softened, about 5 minutes. Set aside. In a large bowl, using a fork, blend crumbled tofu, bread crumbs, peanut butter, soy sauce, Parmesan cheese, carrots, zucchini, parsley, oregano, black pepper and sautéed onion and garlic. Mix well. Using your hands, form mixture into 2-inch balls.

In a large nonstick skillet, heat oil over medium-high heat. When oil is hot, sauté balls, turning frequently, until evenly browned. You may need to do this in several batches, adding oil as needed.

Meatballs can also be baked in a 375° oven for 30 minutes, turning occasionally.

In a medium saucepan, heat tomato sauce over medium heat until heated through. Pour sauce over Tofu Meatballs and serve over Basic Steamed Brown Rice (see recipe, page 242).

Tofu Parmesan

Makes 4 servings • Each serving: 42 grams protein • 9 grams carbohydrate

1½ pounds firm tofu, drained,
  pressed and sliced into
  1 x 3-inch sticks (for directions,
  see "All You Need to Know
  About Tofu," page 10)

2 beaten eggs

1 cup cornmeal

1 cup grated Parmesan cheese

2 teaspoons dried basil

1 teaspoon dried oregano

1 teaspoon dried thyme

freshly ground black pepper,
  to taste

3 tablespoons pure-pressed extra
  virgin olive oil

Prepare tofu and set aside. In a shallow bowl, beat eggs with a fork. In another shallow bowl, using a fork, combine cornmeal, Parmesan cheese, basil, oregano, thyme and black pepper until well blended. Dip tofu sticks in beaten egg, then in cornmeal mixture, coating all sides thoroughly.

In a large nonstick skillet, heat oil over medium-high heat. When oil is hot, add tofu sticks in a single layer and sauté until golden brown on both sides, about 3 to 5 minutes per side. Serve immediately.

Tofu Stroganoff

Makes 4 servings • Each serving: 32 grams protein • 13 grams carbohydrate
1/2 cup Basic Steamed Brown Rice: 3 grams protein • 23 grams carbohydrate
1/2 cup Garlic Mashed Potatoes: 3 grams protein • 26 grams carbohydrate

3 tablespoons pure-pressed extra virgin olive oil

1½ pounds firm tofu, drained, pressed and cut into ½-inch cubes (for directions, see "All You Need to Know About Tofu," page 10)

2 tablespoons unsalted butter

1 medium diced onion

2 minced garlic cloves

3 cups sliced brown or white mushrooms

freshly ground black pepper, to taste

1 tablespoon flour

1 cup whole sour cream

2 tablespoons low-sodium tamari soy sauce

2 teaspoons Dijon mustard

2 tablespoons dry sherry

¼ cup minced fresh parsley

¼ cup slivered fresh basil, or 2 teaspoons dried basil

1 cup fresh green peas or frozen and thawed

In a large nonstick skillet, heat oil over medium-high heat. When oil is hot, add tofu cubes and sauté until browned, stirring occasionally. Remove tofu cubes and set aside.

In the same skillet, melt butter over medium-high heat. When butter is hot and bubbly, add onion and garlic and sauté until softened, about 3 minutes. Reduce heat to medium, add mushrooms and black pepper. Sauté until tender, about 5 to 7 minutes. Sprinkle with flour and sauté 2 minutes. Add sautéed tofu to pan and stir well.

In a small bowl, using a fork, mix sour cream, soy sauce, mustard, sherry, parsley, basil and peas. Stir sauce into vegetable and tofu mixture. Cook over low heat until stroganoff is thickened and heated through, about 10 minutes. Taste, and adjust seasonings. Serve over Basic Steamed Brown Rice (see recipe, page 242) or Garlic Mashed Potatoes (see recipe, page 277).

Vegetarian Chili

Makes 8 servings • Each serving: 19 grams protein • 28 grams carbohydrate

1 cup dried kidney beans; or 28 ounces canned cooked kidney beans, drained and rinsed

3 tablespoons pure-pressed extra virgin olive oil

1 large diced onion

3 minced garlic cloves

1 diced bell pepper

1 cup chopped celery stalks

1 small diced fresh jalapeño pepper; or 1 to 2 tablespoons canned diced green chilies, to taste [wear rubber gloves to prepare fresh jalapeño pepper]

1 tablespoon chili powder

1 tablespoon ground cumin

2 teaspoons dried oregano

⅛ teaspoon cayenne pepper

2 bay leaves

28 ounces chopped canned tomatoes (reserve liquid)

1 cup sliced carrots

1 tablespoon low-sodium tamari soy sauce

freshly ground black pepper, to taste

2 cups vegetable stock (see recipe, page 100), or *low-sodium canned,* or *water*

1 pound firm tofu, drained, pressed and crumbled (for directions, see "All You Need to Know About Tofu," page 10)

2 tablespoons chopped fresh cilantro, for garnish

If using dried beans, soak overnight covering tops of beans with 4 inches of water. Drain beans, cover with fresh water and bring to a boil over high heat. Reduce heat to medium and cook, uncovered until tender, about 45 minutes to 1 hour, stirring occasionally. Drain and set aside.

In a large heavy-bottomed soup pot, heat oil over medium-high heat. When oil is hot, add onion, garlic, bell pepper, celery, jalapeño pepper, chili powder, cumin, oregano, cayenne and bay leaves. Sauté until softened, about 10 minutes.

Add tomatoes and their liquid, carrots, soy sauce, black pepper, vegetable stock or water and kidney beans. Bring to a boil. Reduce heat to low and simmer 30 minutes.

Add crumbled tofu and heat through. Taste, and adjust seasonings. Pour into bowls and sprinkle with cilantro.

Zucchini and Corn Medley

Makes 4 servings • Each serving: 26 grams protein • 17 grams carbohydrate

3 tablespoons unsalted butter

1 medium diced red onion

1 diced red or green bell pepper

*1 pound zucchini, sliced into
    ¼-inch rounds*

*2 cups fresh corn or frozen and
    thawed*

*2 tablespoons fresh slivered basil,
    or 1 teaspoon dried basil*

*2 tablespoons minced fresh
    parsley*

*freshly ground black pepper,
    to taste*

4 eggs

1½ cups whole cottage cheese

*2 tablespoons all-dairy heavy
    cream*

*½ cup grated Monterey Jack
    cheese*

*2 tablespoons grated Parmesan
    cheese, for topping*

Preheat oven to 350°. In a large nonstick skillet, melt butter over medium-high heat. When butter is hot and bubbly, add onion and bell pepper and sauté until softened, about 5 minutes. Add zucchini and corn and sauté another 5 minutes. Add basil, parsley and black pepper and mix well. Remove from heat.

In a large bowl, mix eggs, cottage cheese, cream and Monterey Jack cheese. Add vegetable mixture and mix well. Pour into a greased 2-quart casserole. Top with Parmesan cheese and bake until top is golden and puffy, about 30 to 40 minutes.

Grain, Legume and Rice Side Dishes

Barley

Couscous

Kasha

Legumes

Millet

Polenta

Quinoa

Rice

Risotto

Barley

Barley and Mushroom Casserole

Makes about 4½ cups • Each ⅓ cup serving: 4 grams protein • 22 grams carbohydrate

3 tablespoons unsalted butter

1 small chopped onion

2 cups sliced brown or white mushrooms

1 cup pearl barley, rinsed and drained

3 cups vegetable stock (see recipe, page 100), or *low-sodium canned,* or *water*

freshly ground black pepper, to taste

In a large saucepan with a tight-fitting lid, melt butter over medium-high heat. When butter is hot and bubbly, add onion and sauté until softened, about 5 minutes. Add mushrooms and barley and sauté 5 minutes. Add stock or water, bring to a boil, cover and reduce heat to low. Simmer about 60 to 70 minutes, until all liquid has been absorbed and barley is tender. Season to taste with black pepper.

Couscous

Basic Couscous

Makes about 2½ cups • Each ⅓ cup serving: 2 grams protein • 14 grams carbohydrate

*1 cup vegetable stock
(see recipe, page 100), or
low-sodium canned, or water*

1 tablespoon unsalted butter
1 cup couscous

In a medium saucepan, bring stock and butter to a boil over medium-high heat. In another saucepan, with a tight-fitting lid, pour hot stock over dry couscous. Stir one time, cover and remove from heat. Let stand 10 minutes until all liquid has been absorbed. Fluff with a fork. Serve immediately.

Moroccan Couscous

Makes about 3¹/₄ cups • Each ¹/₃ cup serving: 2 grams protein • 15 grams carbohydrate

1 tablespoon pure-pressed extra virgin olive oil

½ small diced onion

½ diced red bell pepper

1 minced garlic clove

1 cup couscous

1 teaspoon curry powder

1 cup vegetable stock (see recipe, page 100), or low-sodium canned, or water

1 tablespoon unsalted butter

½ cup fresh green peas or frozen and thawed

1 to 2 teaspoons fresh lemon or lime juice

freshly ground black pepper, to taste

dash cayenne pepper

In a medium nonstick skillet, heat oil over medium-high heat. When oil is hot, add onion, bell pepper and garlic. Sauté until softened, about 5 minutes. Add couscous and curry powder and sauté 1 minute.

In a medium saucepan, bring stock, butter, peas, lemon or lime juice, black pepper and cayenne pepper to a boil. Pour hot liquid over couscous, stir once, cover and let sit undisturbed 10 to 15 minutes, until all liquid is absorbed. Fluff with a fork before serving. Taste, and adjust seasonings.

Kasha

Basic Kasha

Makes about 3³/₄ cups • Each ¹/₃ cup serving: 3 grams protein • 14 grams carbohydrate

1½ cups kasha

1 beaten egg

3 cups boiling vegetable stock
(see recipe, page 100), or
low-sodium canned

In a medium saucepan, combine kasha and egg and stir over medium heat until kasha has absorbed all of the egg, and grains are separate and dry-looking, about 3 minutes.

Add boiling stock or water. Cover and simmer over low heat until liquid is absorbed, about 10 to 12 minutes. Remove from heat and let stand, covered, 5 minutes before fluffing with a fork.

Mushroom Kasha Pilaf

Makes about 6¾ cups • Each ⅓ cup serving: 4 grams protein • 16 grams carbohydrate

½ cup chopped raw almonds

2 tablespoons unsalted butter

1 medium diced red onion

2 minced garlic cloves

3 cups sliced brown or white
   mushrooms

1½ cups kasha

1 beaten egg

3 cups boiling vegetable stock
   (see recipe, page 100), or
   low-sodium canned, or water

2 teaspoons low-sodium tamari
   soy sauce

2 tablespoons minced fresh parsley

1 cup fresh green peas, steamed,
   or frozen and thawed

dash cayenne pepper

Put almonds in an ungreased skillet over medium-high heat. Stir or shake pan almost constantly until almonds are evenly browned and toasted. Remove from pan immediately and set aside.

In a large nonstick skillet, melt butter over medium-high heat. When butter is hot and bubbly, add onion and garlic, and sauté until softened, about 5 minutes. Add mushrooms and sauté until tender, about 5 minutes. Set aside.

Mix kasha with beaten egg and pour into a medium saucepan. Cook over medium heat, stirring constantly, until egg is absorbed and grains are separate and dry-looking, about 3 minutes.

Add mushroom-and-onion mixture, stock and soy sauce to kasha mixture. Return to a boil. Reduce heat to low. Cover and simmer until all water is absorbed, about 10 to 12 minutes. Remove from heat and let stand, covered, 5 minutes. Fluff with a fork while adding parsley, peas, chopped almonds and cayenne pepper. Taste, and adjust seasonings.

Legumes

Indian Lentil Dal

Makes about 2¹/₃ cups • Each ¹/₃ cup serving: 7 grams protein • 14 grams carbohydrate

1 cup lentils, picked over and rinsed

3 cups vegetable stock (see recipe, page 100), or low-sodium canned, or water

2 tablespoons unsalted butter

2 tablespoons peeled and finely minced fresh ginger

½ teaspoon cardamom

½ teaspoon ground cumin

½ teaspoon ground turmeric

½ teaspoon red-pepper flakes

2 tablespoons minced fresh cilantro

1 to 2 tablespoons fresh lemon juice, to taste

In a medium saucepan, bring lentils and stock or water to a boil over medium-high heat. Reduce heat to low and simmer, covered, about 30 minutes or until lentils are tender, stirring occasionally.

In a small nonstick skillet, melt butter over medium-high heat. When butter is hot and bubbly, add ginger, cardamom, cumin, turmeric and red-pepper flakes. Sauté until spices are well-coated with butter, about 3 minutes. Add spices, cilantro and lemon juice to cooked lentils. Simmer 10 minutes over low heat. Taste, and adjust seasonings.

Mexican-Style Beans

Makes about 5½ cups • Each ⅓ cup serving: 5 grams protein • 15 grams carbohydrate

2 tablespoons pure-pressed
  extra virgin olive oil

½ cup chopped onion

2 minced garlic cloves

1 diced green or red bell pepper

1 small diced fresh jalapeño
  pepper; or 1 to 2 tablespoons
  canned diced green chilies, to
  taste [wear rubber gloves to
  prepare fresh pepper]

2 teaspoons ground cumin

2 teaspoons dried oregano

1 tablespoon minced fresh cilantro

4 cups cooked and drained black
  beans or pinto beans

1 cup Basic Tomato Sauce or
  Enchilada Sauce, (see recipes,
  pages 300 and 305); or store-
  bought (no sugar added)

freshly ground black pepper,
  to taste

Topping

whole sour cream   grated Monterey Jack cheese

In a large nonstick skillet, heat oil over medium-high heat. When oil is hot, add onion, garlic, bell pepper, jalapeño pepper, cumin, oregano and cilantro, and sauté until vegetables are softened and nearly tender, about 5 minutes.

Add drained beans, enchilada sauce or tomato sauce and black pepper and stir well. Bring to a boil, reduce heat to medium and cook, stirring occasionally, about 10 minutes. Taste, and adjust seasonings. Serve with a tablespoon each of sour cream and grated cheese.

Middle Eastern Lentils
with Vegetables

Makes about 6¼ cups • Each ⅓ cup serving: 6 grams protein • 13 grams carbohydrate

1½ cups dried lentils, picked over
    and rinsed

3 cups water

2 tablespoons pure-pressed extra
    virgin olive oil

1 medium chopped onion

2 minced garlic cloves

1 diced bell pepper

2 chopped celery stalks

2 diced carrots

1 medium zucchini, cut into
    ¼-inch half rounds

1 bay leaf

1 teaspoon ground cumin

1 teaspoon dried oregano

2 tablespoons minced fresh parsley

freshly ground black pepper,
    to taste

1 to 2 tablespoons fresh lemon
    juice, to taste

Rinse and drain lentils. In a Dutch oven or deep saucepan, cover lentils with water and bring to a boil. Reduce heat, cover and cook until lentils are almost tender, about 20 minutes.

While lentils are cooking, heat oil in a large nonstick skillet over medium-high heat. When oil is hot, add onion, garlic and bell pepper and sauté until softened, about 5 minutes. Add celery, carrots, zucchini, bay leaf, cumin, oregano, parsley and black pepper, and sauté 5 more minutes. Add vegetable mixture to lentils and mix well.

Cover and cook until lentils and vegetables are tender, about 15 minutes, adding more water to pot if needed. Add lemon juice. Taste, and adjust seasonings.

Millet

Basic Millet

Makes about 3½ cups • Each ⅓ cup serving: 3 grams protein • 20 grams carbohydrate

1 tablespoon unsalted butter
1 cup millet, rinsed and
drained

3 cups vegetable stock (see recipe,
page 100), or *low-sodium*
canned, or *water*

In a medium saucepan, melt butter over medium-high heat. When butter is hot and bubbly, add millet and cook over medium heat, stirring until lightly browned, about 2 minutes.

Add stock or water. Return to a boil, cover, reduce heat to low and simmer about 30 minutes or until all liquid has been absorbed. Remove from heat and let stand 5 minutes before fluffing with a fork.

Curried Millet

Makes about 4½ cups • Each ⅓ cup serving: 4 grams protein • 21 grams carbohydrate

2 tablespoons unsalted butter

1 cup millet, rinsed and drained

1 small diced onion

2 minced garlic cloves

2 teaspoons peeled and finely
minced fresh ginger

1 teaspoon curry powder

1 teaspoon ground cumin

1 teaspoon ground coriander

1 teaspoon ground turmeric

dash cayenne pepper

3 cups vegetable stock
(see recipe, page 100), or
low-sodium canned, or water

1 cup fresh green peas steamed,
or frozen and thawed

1 tablespoon fresh lime juice

In a medium saucepan, melt butter over medium-high heat. When butter is hot and bubbly, add millet, onion, garlic, ginger, curry powder, cumin, coriander, turmeric and cayenne pepper. Sauté until well mixed and onion is softened, about 5 minutes.

Add vegetable stock or water. Bring to a boil. Reduce heat to low, cover and simmer until all liquid is absorbed, about 30 minutes. Remove from heat and let stand 5 minutes. Stir in peas and lime juice while fluffing with a fork.

Polenta

Basic Polenta

Makes about 3⅓ cups • Each ⅓ cup serving: 8 grams protein • 53 grams carbohydrate

*4 cups vegetable stock (see recipe,
  page 100), or low-sodium
  canned, or water*

1 cup polenta
⅓ cup grated Parmesan cheese
3 tablespoons unsalted butter

In a large saucepan, bring stock or water to a boil. Slowly drizzle in polenta in a steady stream, stirring constantly. Reduce heat to medium-low and continue cooking, stirring frequently, until mixture thickens, about 15 to 20 minutes. Stir in Parmesan cheese and butter and serve immediately.

Polenta and Mushrooms

Makes about 4⅓ cups • Each ⅓ cup serving: 8 grams protein • 53 grams carbohydrate

2 tablespoons unsalted butter

1 cup diced onion

2 cups sliced brown or white
  mushrooms

freshly ground black pepper,
  to taste

4 cups vegetable stock (see recipe,
  page 100), or low-sodium
  canned, or water

1 cup polenta

⅓ cup grated Parmesan cheese

In a large nonstick skillet, melt butter over medium-high heat. When butter is hot and bubbly, add onion and sauté until softened, about 5 minutes. Add mushrooms and sauté until tender, about 5 minutes. Season to taste with black pepper. Set aside.

In a deep saucepan, bring stock or water to a boil. Slowly sprinkle in polenta, whisking constantly to avoid lumps. Cook over medium heat, stirring, until mixture thickens and bubbles, about 15 to 20 minutes. Add onion and mushroom mixture and Parmesan cheese and mix well.

Polenta Variations

Grilled Polenta: Prepare Basic Polenta (see recipe, page 237). Pour cooked polenta into a greased 9 x 9-inch pan and spread evenly across pan. Cool until hardened. Remove from pan and cut into squares or triangles. Place on a greased baking sheet and broil until browned and crisp on both sides. Brush with compound butter before serving (see Compound Butters, page 288).

Makes about 3¹/₃ cups • Each ¹/₃ cup serving: 8 grams protein • 53 grams carbohydrate

Polenta with Fresh Basil and Ricotta Cheese: Prepare Basic Polenta (see recipe, page 237). Add 2 tablespoons slivered fresh basil and 1 cup whole ricotta cheese as mixture thickens.

Makes about 4¹/₃ cups • Each ¹/₃ cup serving: 10 grams protein • 54 grams carbohydrate

Polenta with Gorgonzola Cheese: Prepare Basic Polenta (see recipe, page 237), substituting ½ cup crumbled Gorgonzola cheese for the Parmesan cheese, and adding ¼ cup slivered fresh basil, *or* 2 teaspoons dried basil.

Makes about 3¹/₂ cups • Each ¹/₃ cup serving: 10 grams protein • 53 grams carbohydrate

Polenta with Sun-Dried Tomato Pesto: Prepare Basic Polenta, (see recipe, page 237), adding ½ cup Sun-Dried Tomato Pesto (see recipe, page 295).

Makes about 3³/₄ cups • Each ¹/₃ cup serving: 9 grams protein • 54 grams carbohydrate

Quinoa

Quinoa (pronounced KEEN-WAA) is a grain high in thiamin, iron, vitamin B$_6$ and phosphorus. It was a primary food of Native Americans over five thousand years ago and a staple of the Incan civilization.

Basic Quinoa

Makes about 3 cups • Each ⅓ cup serving: 3 grams protein • 14 grams carbohydrate

2 cups vegetable stock (see recipe, page 100), or low-sodium canned, or water

1 cup quinoa, rinsed and drained

In a medium saucepan with a tight-fitting lid, bring stock or water to a boil. Add quinoa and return to a boil. Cover, reduce heat to low and simmer 15 minutes until all liquid has been absorbed. Remove from heat and let sit, covered and undisturbed, for 10 minutes. Fluff with a fork before serving.

Quinoa with Spinach and Feta Cheese

Makes about 5³/₄ cups • Each ¹/₃ cup serving: 5 grams protein • 15 grams carbohydrate

2 cups vegetable stock
  (see recipe, page 100), or
  low-sodium canned, or water

1 cup quinoa, rinsed and drained

1 bunch spinach equal to about
  1 cup cooked spinach, well
  drained and chopped; or
  8 ounces packaged frozen
  spinach, thawed, drained and
  chopped

2 tablespoons pure-pressed extra
  virgin olive oil

2 minced garlic cloves

½ cup diced onion

1 cup chopped tomatoes

¼ cup slivered fresh basil, or
  2 teaspoons dried basil

1 teaspoon grated lemon zest

½ cup crumbled feta cheese

freshly ground black pepper,
  to taste

In a medium saucepan with a tight-fitting lid, bring stock or water to a boil. Add quinoa and return to a boil. Cover, reduce heat to low and simmer 15 minutes until all liquid has been absorbed. Remove from heat and let sit, covered and undisturbed, for 10 minutes. Set aside.

Wash spinach well, removing stems. With water still clinging to leaves, place in a medium saucepan with a tight-fitting lid. Turn heat to medium-high and steam until leaves are wilted, about 2 to 3 minutes. Drain in a colander, pressing out all liquid with the back of a wooden spoon. Chop coarsely and set aside.

In a large nonstick skillet, heat oil over medium-high heat. When oil is hot, add garlic and onion and sauté until softened, about 5 minutes. Add tomatoes and cook 5 minutes. Add spinach, basil, prepared quinoa, lemon zest, feta cheese and black pepper. Mix well and cook until heated through. Taste, and adjust seasonings.

Rice

Basic Steamed Brown Rice

Makes about 3 cups • Each ⅓ cup serving: 2 grams protein • 16 grams carbohydrate

1 tablespoon unsalted butter

1 cup long-grain brown rice,
  rinsed and drained

2 cups vegetable stock (see recipe,
  page 100), or low-sodium
  canned, or water

In a medium saucepan with a tight-fitting lid, melt butter over medium-high heat. When butter is hot and bubbly, add drained rice and sauté until grains are dried and separate. Add vegetable stock or water and bring to a boil. Cover, reduce heat to low and simmer undisturbed about 45 to 50 minutes, until all the liquid is absorbed. Remove pan from heat and let sit, covered, 10 minutes. Fluff rice with a fork and serve.

Brown Rice Pilaf

Makes about 5 cups • Each ⅓ cup serving: 5 grams protein • 25 grams carbohydrate

½ cup long-grain brown rice, rinsed and drained

¼ cup wild rice, rinsed and drained

¼ cup wheat berries, rinsed and drained

2 cups vegetable stock (see recipe, page 100), or low-sodium canned, or water

2 tablespoons pure-pressed extra virgin olive oil

1 small diced onion

1 minced garlic clove

2 diced celery stalks

1 diced red or green bell pepper

1 teaspoon ground cumin

1 teaspoon chili powder

1 teaspoon dried oregano

1 cup sliced brown or white mushrooms

freshly ground black pepper, to taste

½ cup fresh green peas or frozen and thawed

In a large saucepan with a tight-fitting lid, bring brown rice, wild rice, wheat berries and stock to a boil. Cover, reduce heat to low and simmer until all liquid is absorbed, about 45 to 50 minutes. Remove from heat and let sit, covered and undisturbed, for 10 minutes.

In a large nonstick skillet, heat oil over medium-high heat. When oil is hot, add onion, garlic, celery, bell pepper, cumin, chili powder and oregano, and sauté until softened, about 6 minutes, stirring occasionally. Add mushrooms and black pepper and sauté 5 minutes. Stir in peas and cook until heated through.

Combine sautéed vegetables with cooked grains. Mix well, stirring with a fork or wooden spoon. Taste, and adjust seasonings.

Brown Rice with Mushrooms

Makes about 6 cups • Each ⅓ serving: 3 grams protein • 17 grams carbohydrate

½ cup sliced raw almonds, for
   garnish

2 tablespoons unsalted butter

2 minced garlic cloves

1½ cups long-grain brown rice,
   rinsed and drained

3 cups thinly sliced brown or
   white mushrooms

1 tablespoon low-sodium tamari
   soy sauce

freshly ground black pepper,
   to taste

3 cups vegetable stock (see recipe,
   page 100), or low-sodium
   canned, or water

2 tablespoons minced fresh
   parsley, for garnish

Put almonds in an ungreased skillet over medium-high heat. Stir nuts or shake pan almost constantly until almonds are evenly browned and toasted. Remove from pan immediately and set aside.

Melt butter over medium-high heat in a medium saucepan with a tight-fitting lid. When butter is hot and bubbly, add garlic and rice and sauté about 3 minutes. Add mushrooms, soy sauce and black pepper and sauté 3 minutes. Add stock or water and bring to a boil. Cover tightly, reduce heat to low and simmer 45 minutes. Remove from heat and let sit, covered and undisturbed, for 10 minutes. Remove lid and fluff rice with a fork. Taste, and adjust seasonings. Spoon into a serving bowl and sprinkle with almonds and parsley.

Greek Rice

Makes 6 cups • Each ⅓ cup serving: 3 grams protein • 16 grams carbohydrate

2 tablespoons pure-pressed extra
  virgin olive oil

1 small diced yellow onion

1 minced garlic clove

1½ cups long-grain brown rice,
  rinsed and drained

3 cups vegetable stock (see recipe,
  page 100), or low-sodium
  canned, or water

3 tablespoons fresh lemon juice

2 teaspoons dried oregano

⅓ cup diced Kalamata olives

⅓ cup minced fresh parsley

freshly ground black pepper,
  to taste

½ cup crumbled feta cheese

In a medium saucepan with a tight-fitting lid, heat oil over medium-high heat. When oil is hot, add onion and garlic and sauté until softened, about 5 minutes. Add rice and sauté 2 minutes, stirring occasionally. Add stock or water. Bring to a boil. Cover and reduce heat to low. Simmer 45 to 50 minutes. Remove from heat and let sit, covered and undisturbed, for 10 minutes. Remove lid and fluff rice with a fork. Add lemon juice, oregano, Kalamata olives, parsley and black pepper. Stir in feta cheese and mix well. Taste, and adjust seasonings.

Green Onion and Lime Rice

Makes about 6 cups • Each ⅓ cup serving: 4 grams protein • 17 grams carbohydrate

¾ cup slivered raw almonds, for
  garnish

1½ cups long-grain brown rice,
  rinsed and drained

3 cups vegetable stock (see recipe,
  page 100), or low-sodium
  canned, or water

¾ cup minced fresh parsley

½ cup finely slivered scallions

1 tablespoon pure-pressed sesame
  oil

2 tablespoons fresh lime juice

grated zest of 1 large lime

Put almonds in an ungreased skillet over medium-high heat. Stir nuts or shake pan almost constantly until almonds are evenly browned and toasted. Remove from pan immediately and set aside.

In a medium saucepan with a tight-fitting lid, bring rice and stock or water to a boil. Cover and reduce heat to low. Simmer 45 to 50 minutes. Set aside and let sit undisturbed and covered for 10 minutes. Remove lid and fluff rice with a fork. Stir in parsley, scallions, sesame oil, lime juice and lime zest. Sprinkle top with toasted almonds.

Indian Rice

Makes about 6¼ cups • Each ⅓ cup serving: 3 grams protein • 17 grams carbohydrate

¾ cup coarsely chopped raw
cashews, for garnish

3 tablespoons unsalted butter

2 teaspoons peeled and finely
minced fresh ginger

1 cup diced carrots

1½ cups long-grain brown rice,
rinsed and drained

1 teaspoon ground cardamom

1 teaspoon curry powder

2 whole cinnamon sticks, broken
into pieces

2 cups vegetable stock
(see recipe, page 100), or
low-sodium canned, or water

1 cup coconut milk

Put cashews in an ungreased skillet over medium-high heat. Stir nuts or shake pan almost constantly, until cashews are evenly browned and toasted. Remove from pan immediately and set aside.

In a medium saucepan with a tight-fitting lid, melt butter over medium-high heat. When butter is hot and bubbly, add ginger, carrots, rice, cardamom, curry powder, and cinnamon sticks and sauté over medium heat about 5 minutes. Add stock or water and coconut milk, and bring to a boil. Lower heat, cover pot and simmer 45 to 50 minutes.

Remove from heat and let sit, covered and undisturbed, for 10 minutes. Remove lid, fluff with a fork and discard cinnamon sticks. Taste, and adjust seasonings. Transfer to a serving bowl and sprinkle with cashews.

Spinach Rice Pilaf

Makes about 4½ cups • Each ⅓ cup serving: 3 grams protein • 16 grams carbohydrate

⅓ cup coarsely chopped raw
  almonds, for garnish

1 bunch spinach equal to about
  1 cup cooked spinach, well
  drained and chopped; or
  8 ounces packaged frozen
  spinach, thawed, drained
  and chopped

2 tablespoons unsalted butter

¼ cup minced red onion

1 cup long-grain brown rice,
  rinsed and drained

2 cups vegetable stock (see recipe,
  page 100), or low-sodium
  canned, or water

freshly ground black pepper,
  to taste

dash cayenne pepper

Put almonds in an ungreased skillet over medium-high heat. Stir
nuts or shake pan almost constantly until almonds are evenly
browned and toasted. Remove from pan immediately and set aside.

Wash spinach well, removing stems. With water still clinging to
leaves, place in a medium saucepan with a tight-fitting lid. Turn heat
to medium-high and steam until leaves are wilted, about 2 to 3 minutes. Drain in a colander, pressing out all liquid with the back of a
wooden spoon. Chop coarsely and set aside.

In a medium saucepan, melt butter over medium-high heat. When
butter is hot and bubbly, add onion and sauté until softened, about 5
minutes. Add brown rice and sauté 2 minutes. Stir in stock or water
and bring to a boil. Reduce heat to low and simmer 45 to 50 minutes,
until all liquid is absorbed. Remove from heat and let sit, covered and
undisturbed, for 10 minutes. Remove lid, fluff with a fork and stir in
cooked spinach, black pepper and cayenne pepper. Mix well. Taste,
and adjust seasonings. Transfer to a serving bowl and sprinkle with
chopped almonds.

Tomato Vegetable Rice

Makes about 7³/₄ cups • Each ¹/₃ cup serving: 3 grams protein • 17 grams carbohydrate

2 tablespoons unsalted butter

1 tablespoon pure-pressed extra virgin olive oil

1 diced green bell pepper

1 medium diced red onion

2 minced garlic cloves

2 diced celery stalks

1 teaspoon ground cumin

1 teaspoon dried oregano

1½ cups long-grain brown rice, rinsed and drained

1½ cups diced tomatoes

3 cups vegetable stock (see recipe, page 100), or *low-sodium canned,* or *water*

freshly ground black pepper, to taste

1 cup fresh green peas, or frozen and thawed

2 tablespoons minced fresh parsley

¼ cup chopped black or green olives

In a medium saucepan with a tight-fitting lid, heat butter and oil over medium-high heat. When hot, add green pepper, onion, garlic, celery, cumin and oregano. Sauté until softened, about 5 minutes. Add rice and sauté until coated with butter and oil, about 2 minutes. Add tomatoes, stock or water and black pepper and stir well.

Bring to a boil. Cover tightly and reduce heat to simmer. Simmer 45 minutes, until all liquid is absorbed. Remove from heat and let sit, covered and undisturbed, for 10 minutes. Remove lid and fluff rice with a fork. Stir in peas, parsley and olives. Taste, and adjust seasonings.

Risotto

Risotto with Asparagus, Sun-Dried Tomatoes and Feta Cheese

Makes about 7 cups • Each ⅓ cup serving: 4 grams protein • 17 grams carbohydrate

3 tablespoons pure-pressed extra virgin olive oil, or oil from sun-dried tomatoes

2 minced garlic cloves

1 small diced onion

½ cup sun-dried tomatoes, drained and slivered

1½ cups long-grain brown rice, rinsed and drained

4 cups vegetable stock (see recipe, page 100), or low-sodium canned, simmering hot

½ pound asparagus, tough ends trimmed, cut into ½-inch pieces

¼ cup slivered fresh basil, or 2 teaspoons dried basil

1 cup crumbled feta cheese

1 tablespoon fresh lemon juice

2 teaspoons grated lemon zest

freshly ground black pepper, to taste

In a large saucepan, heat oil over medium-high heat. When oil is hot, add garlic and onion and sauté until softened, about 5 minutes. Add sun-dried tomatoes and brown rice. Stir gently to thoroughly coat grains with oil.

Ladle 1 cup of simmering hot stock into rice, stir well and cook over medium heat, uncovered, stirring constantly until all liquid is absorbed. Add another cup of hot stock and stir constantly until all liquid is absorbed. Continue adding one cup at a time, until all of stock has been absorbed and rice is tender. (Adding stock cup by cup will take about 20 to 30 minutes.)

Cook asparagus until just barely tender by immersing into boiling water about 3 to 6 minutes. Drain, rinse under cold water and drain again.

After all stock has been added and rice is cooked to your liking, add asparagus pieces, basil, feta cheese, lemon juice, grated lemon zest and black pepper. Taste, and adjust seasonings.

Nonstarchy Vegetable
Side Dishes

Baked Spinach and Feta-Filled Tomatoes

Makes 4 side-dish servings • Each serving: 10 grams protein • 13 grams carbohydrate

2 firm large tomatoes

1 bunch spinach equal to about 1 cup cooked spinach, well drained and chopped; or 8 ounces packaged frozen spinach, thawed, drained and chopped

2 tablespoons unsalted butter

1 minced garlic clove

1 small diced red onion

½ cup crumbled feta cheese

½ cup fresh or dried whole-grain bread crumbs

1 tablespoon Dijon mustard

2 tablespoons slivered fresh basil, or 2 teaspoons dried basil

1 beaten egg

freshly ground black pepper, to taste

dash cayenne pepper

1 tablespoon grated Parmesan cheese

4 raw walnut halves, for garnish

Preheat oven to 350°. Cut tomatoes in half crosswise, scoop out pulp and seeds, leaving shell intact.

Wash spinach well, removing stems. With water still clinging to leaves, place in a medium saucepan with a tight-fitting lid. Turn heat to medium-high and steam until leaves are wilted, 2 to 3 minutes. Drain in a colander, pressing out all liquid with the back of a wooden spoon. Chop coarsely and set aside.

In a small nonstick skillet, melt butter over medium-high heat. When butter is hot and bubbly, add garlic and onion and sauté until softened, about 5 minutes. Remove from heat and set aside.

In a medium bowl, using a fork, combine prepared spinach, feta cheese, bread crumbs, mustard, basil, egg, black pepper, cayenne pepper, sautéed onion and garlic. Mix well. Mound filling into each tomato half. Sprinkle with Parmesan cheese and set on a lightly greased baking sheet. Bake about 20 minutes or until filling is heated through. Garnish with a whole walnut half.

Bell Pepper Medley

Makes 4 side-dish servings. Each serving: 2 grams protein • trace carbohydrate

3 tablespoons pure-pressed extra
 virgin olive oil

4 bell peppers (any combination
 of red, green or yellow), cut
 into slivers

1 minced garlic clove

freshly ground black pepper,
 to taste

1 tablespoon balsamic vinegar

2 tablespoons rinsed and drained
 capers (optional)

2 tablespoons crumbled feta
 cheese

In a large nonstick skillet, heat oil over medium-high heat. When oil is hot, add bell peppers and garlic and sauté until softened and tender, about 10 minutes, stirring occasionally.

Remove from heat. Add black pepper, balsamic vinegar, capers and feta cheese. Toss gently. Taste, and adjust seasonings. Serve at room temperature.

Broiled Eggplant

Makes 4 side-dish servings • Each serving: 7 grams protein • 4 grams carbohydrate

1 large eggplant, (peeled,
  if desired)

¼ cup pure-pressed extra virgin
  olive oil

1½ cups Basic Tomato Sauce or
  Basil Pesto (see recipes, pages 300
  and 294); or store-bought

1 teaspoon dried oregano

1 teaspoon dried basil

freshly ground black pepper,
  to taste

½ cup grated Parmesan cheese,
  for topping

Preheat broiler. Slice eggplant into ½-inch-thick rounds. Lightly oil a baking sheet.

Using a pastry brush, brush one side of eggplant rounds with olive oil. Arrange in a single layer, olive-oil side up, on baking sheet. Broil about 10 minutes about 4 inches from the heat. Turn slices and spread tomato sauce or pesto on top side of eggplant. Sprinkle with oregano, basil and black pepper. Broil about 5 to 10 minutes until eggplant is tender. Sprinkle with Parmesan cheese and serve hot.

Creamed Spinach with Mushrooms

Makes 4 side-dish servings • Each serving: 3 grams protein • 3 grams carbohydrate

2 bunches spinach equal to about
  2 cups cooked spinach, well
  drained and chopped; or
  16 ounces packaged frozen
  spinach, thawed, drained
  and chopped

2 tablespoons unsalted butter

2 tablespoons chopped red onion

2 cups thinly sliced brown or
  white mushrooms

1 teaspoon grated lemon zest

freshly ground black pepper,
  to taste

2 tablespoons unsalted butter

1 tablespoon flour

1 teaspoon Dijon mustard

½ cup all-dairy heavy cream,
  heated to simmering

Wash spinach well, removing stems. With water still clinging to leaves, place in a medium saucepan with a tight-fitting lid. Turn heat to medium-high and steam until leaves are wilted, about 2 to 3 minutes. Drain in a colander, pressing out all liquid with the back of a wooden spoon. Chop fine and set aside.

In a large nonstick skillet, melt 2 tablespoons butter over medium-high heat. When butter is hot and bubbly, add onion and mushrooms and sauté until softened, about 5 minutes. Add lemon zest and season to taste with black pepper. Remove from pan and set aside.

Melt remaining 2 tablespoons butter in same skillet. Add flour and mustard and cook 2 minutes over medium heat, stirring constantly. Whisk in the hot cream and stir until smooth and thickened. Add chopped spinach, onion and mushrooms and stir well. Cook until heated through. Taste, and adjust seasonings.

Crustless Zucchini Quiche

Makes 8 side-dish servings • Each serving: 13 grams protein • trace carbohydrate

2 tablespoons pure-pressed extra
   virgin olive oil

½ cup minced red onion

1 minced garlic clove

2 pounds zucchini, sliced into
   thin rounds

4 eggs

1 cup all-dairy heavy cream

¼ cup chopped fresh parsley

2 teaspoons dried oregano

4 ounces canned diced chilies

2 cups grated Monterey Jack
   cheese

freshly ground black pepper,
   to taste

Preheat oven to 350°. In a large skillet, heat oil over medium-high heat. When oil is hot, add onion and garlic and sauté until softened, about 5 minutes. Add sliced zucchini and sauté 5 minutes until barely tender.

In a large bowl, using a fork, whisk eggs and cream until well blended. Stir in zucchini and onion mixture, parsley, oregano, chilies, Monterey Jack cheese and black pepper. Mix well. Spoon into a greased oven-proof casserole or 9-inch pie pan and bake about 40 minutes, or until egg custard is set in center. A knife inserted into the center of the quiche should come out clean. Let sit 10 minutes before slicing.

Curried Cauliflower

Makes 4 side-dish servings • Each serving: 4 grams protein • 3 grams carbohydrate

1 cup water

*1 large head cauliflower,
separated into florets*

2 tablespoons unsalted butter

*2 tablespoons pure-pressed
monounsaturated vegetable oil*

1 large diced onion

1 teaspoon mustard seeds

2 minced garlic cloves

*2 teaspoons peeled and finely
minced fresh ginger*

1 teaspoon ground coriander

1 teaspoon ground cumin

1 teaspoon turmeric

1 teaspoon curry powder

*freshly ground black pepper,
to taste*

dash cayenne pepper

*1 tablespoon fresh lemon or lime
juice*

1 cup whole plain yogurt

*1 tablespoon chopped fresh
cilantro, for garnish*

In a large saucepan, bring water to a boil. Add cauliflower florets and cook until barely tender, about 5 minutes. Drain and set aside.

In a large nonstick skillet, heat butter and oil over medium-high heat. When hot, add onion and sauté until softened, about 5 minutes. Add mustard seeds and stir until seeds begin to pop, about 1 minute.

Add garlic, ginger, coriander, cumin, turmeric, curry powder, black pepper and cayenne pepper. Stir and cook until well mixed, about 2 minutes. Reduce heat to low. Add lemon or lime juice and yogurt, and mix well. Add cooked cauliflower. Stir until well blended and evenly coated with curry spices. Taste, and adjust seasonings. Sprinkle with chopped cilantro before serving.

Green Beans in Peanut Sauce

Makes 4 side-dish servings • Each serving: 6 grams protein • 4 grams carbohydrate

1 pound fresh green beans, ends trimmed, and sliced diagonally into 1-inch pieces

3 tablespoons organic peanut butter, smooth or chunky (no honey or sugar added)

1 cup vegetable stock (see recipe, page 100), or low-sodium canned, or water

1 minced garlic clove

2 teaspoons peeled and finely minced fresh ginger

1 tablespoon fresh lime juice

¼ teaspoon cayenne pepper

1 tablespoon low-sodium tamari soy sauce

1 tablespoon minced fresh cilantro, for garnish

Cook green beans in boiling water until just tender, about 5 minutes or more. Drain and set aside.

In a small saucepan, bring peanut butter, stock or water, garlic, ginger, lime juice, cayenne pepper and soy sauce to a boil. Reduce heat and simmer 5 minutes. Taste, and adjust seasonings.

Pour sauce over green beans. Sprinkle with cilantro and serve immediately.

Green Beans with Sesame Mayonnaise

Makes 4 side-dish servings • Each serving: 1 gram protein • 1 gram carbohydrate

*1 tablespoon raw sesame seeds
for garnish*

*1 pound fresh green beans,
ends trimmed*

*⅓ cup mayonnaise (made from
pure-pressed oil)*

2 tablespoons whole sour cream

2 teaspoons fresh lime juice

*½ teaspoon pure-pressed sesame
oil*

*freshly ground black pepper,
to taste*

dash cayenne pepper

Put sesame seeds in an ungreased skillet over medium-high heat. Shake pan or stir seeds almost constantly until seeds are evenly browned and toasted and begin to pop. Remove from pan immediately and set aside.

Cook green beans in boiling water until just tender, about 5 minutes or more. Drain well and arrange on a serving platter.

In a small bowl, using a fork, mix mayonnaise, sour cream, lime juice, sesame oil, black pepper and cayenne pepper until well blended. Taste, and adjust seasonings.

Pour sauce over green beans and sprinkle with sesame seeds. Serve at room temperature.

Indonesian Asparagus

Makes 4 side-dish servings • Each serving: 6 grams protein • 2 grams carbohydrate

2 tablespoons pure-pressed
   peanut oil

½ cup chopped red onion

1 teaspoon dried cardamom

½ teaspoon red-pepper flakes

2 teaspoons ground coriander

2 teaspoons peeled and finely
   minced fresh ginger

2 tablespoons creamy organic
   peanut butter (no honey or
   sugar added)

2 tablespoons fresh lime juice

1 can (14 ounces) coconut milk

1 tablespoon minced fresh
   cilantro

1 tablespoon chopped scallions

freshly ground black pepper,
   to taste

2 pounds fresh asparagus
   (tough ends trimmed), cut
   into 1½-inch pieces

In a large nonstick skillet, heat oil over medium-high heat. When oil is hot, add onion and sauté until softened, about 5 minutes. Add cardamom, red-pepper flakes, coriander, ginger, peanut butter, lime juice, coconut milk, cilantro, scallions and black pepper. Mix well. Bring to a boil, reduce heat to low and simmer 2 minutes.

Add asparagus and cook until tender, 3 to 6 minutes. Taste, and adjust seasonings. Serve immediately.

Italian Cauliflower

Makes 4 side-dish servings • Each serving: 4 grams protein • 3 grams carbohydrate

*1 large head cauliflower,
  separated into florets*

*1 cup Basic Tomato Sauce
  (see recipe, page 300), or
  store-bought*

*2 teaspoons rinsed and
  drained capers*

¼ cup chopped green olives

*freshly ground black pepper,
  to taste*

*2 tablespoons grated Parmesan
  cheese, for garnish*

*1 tablespoon minced fresh
  parsley, for garnish*

In a large saucepan, bring water to a boil. Add cauliflower florets and steam until barely tender, about 5 minutes. Drain and set aside.

In a medium saucepan, heat tomato sauce over medium heat until simmering hot. Add capers, green olives, cauliflower and black pepper. Cook until heated through. Taste, and adjust seasonings. Garnish with Parmesan cheese and parsley and serve immediately.

Piperade
(Bell Pepper and Tomato Stew)

Makes 6 side-dish servings • Each serving: 2 grams protein • 2 grams carbohydrate

2 tablespoons pure-pressed extra
  virgin olive oil

1 large onion, sliced into thin
  slivers

1 minced garlic clove

2 red bell peppers, cut into thin
  slivers

2 green bell peppers, cut into thin
  slivers

4 large tomatoes, peeled, seeded
  and chopped*

2 tablespoons slivered fresh basil,
  or 2 teaspoons dried basil

¼ teaspoon red-pepper flakes

freshly ground black pepper,
  to taste

In a large nonstick skillet, heat oil over medium-high heat. When oil is hot, add onion, garlic and bell peppers and sauté over medium heat until softened, about 5 minutes.

Add tomatoes, basil, red-pepper flakes and black pepper. Cook uncovered over medium heat, stirring occasionally, until mixture thickens and most of tomato liquid has evaporated, about 30 minutes. Taste, and adjust seasonings.

---

*To peel and seed tomatoes: Plunge tomatoes into boiling water for about 20 seconds, then into cold water. Skins will slip off easily. Cut tomatoes in half and gently squeeze. Scoop out seeds with a small spoon or your fingers.

Ratatouille

Makes 6 side-dish servings • Each serving: 4 grams protein • 3 grams carbohydrate

3 tablespoons pure-pressed extra virgin olive oil

1 large chopped onion

3 minced garlic cloves

1 large eggplant, (peeled, if desired) and cut into ½-inch cubes

1 red bell pepper, cut into ½-inch pieces

1 green bell pepper, cut into ½-inch pieces

1 large zucchini, cut into ¼-inch half circles

1 cup green beans, ends trimmed, and sliced diagonally into 1-inch pieces

6 chopped ripe large tomatoes

2 tablespoons tomato paste

¼ cup chopped fresh parsley

¼ cup red wine

½ cup water

2 tablespoons slivered fresh basil, or 2 teaspoons dried basil

½ teaspoon dried thyme

½ teaspoon dried rosemary

½ teaspoon dried marjoram

1 bay leaf

1 tablespoon balsamic vinegar

finely ground black pepper, to taste

In a large Dutch oven or flameproof casserole, heat oil over medium-high heat. When oil is hot, add onion and garlic and sauté until softened, about 5 minutes.

Add eggplant and bell peppers and cook until softened, about 8 more minutes. Add zucchini, green beans, tomatoes, tomato paste, parsley, wine, water and herbs. Mix well. Bring to a boil, reduce heat and simmer, uncovered, 20 minutes, stirring occasionally.

Add balsamic vinegar and black pepper. Taste, and adjust seasonings. Simmer 15 more minutes. Serve hot, warm or cold.

Roasted Pepper Medley

Makes 6 side-dish servings • Each serving: trace protein • trace carbohydrate

6 assorted peppers; red, yellow, green and pasilla

¼ cup pure-pressed extra virgin olive oil

2 minced garlic cloves

2 tablespoons balsamic vinegar

1 tablespoon Dijon mustard

freshly ground black pepper, to taste

Roast peppers directly over a gas flame, or under preheated broiler on a broiler rack. Using tongs, turn peppers frequently until blistered and blackened on all sides. Place peppers in a bowl with a plate on top. Let steam for 15 minutes to loosen skins. Peel off all charred skin. Discard skin along with seeds. Cut roasted flesh into slivers.

In a small bowl, using a fork, mix olive oil, garlic, balsamic vinegar, mustard and black pepper until well blended. Pour over peppers and marinate at least 15 minutes before serving at room temperature.

Sautéed Mixed Squash with Cumin and Chili Powder

Makes 4 side-dish servings • Each serving: 2 grams protein • trace carbohydrate

4 small crookneck yellow squash, cut into ¼-inch rounds

4 small zucchini, cut into ¼-inch rounds

2 tablespoons pure-pressed extra virgin olive oil

2 minced garlic cloves

1 teaspoon chili powder

1 teaspoon ground cumin

1 teaspoon dried oregano

freshly ground black pepper, to taste

2 tablespoons fresh lime juice

In a medium saucepan, boil 1 cup water. Add squash and zucchini and cook until barely tender, stirring occasionally, 3 to 5 minutes. Using a slotted spoon, remove squash from pan and drain well. Set aside.

In a large nonstick skillet, heat oil over medium-high heat. When oil is hot, add garlic, chili powder, cumin, oregano and black pepper. Sauté until spices are well-coated with oil.

Add reserved squash and lime juice and toss gently until well-coated with spices and heated through. Taste, and adjust seasonings.

Sautéed Mushrooms

Makes 4 side-dish servings • Each serving: 3 grams protein • 2 grams carbohydrate

3 tablespoons unsalted butter

¼ cup chopped scallions

1 pound thickly sliced brown or
  white mushrooms

2 teaspoons low-sodium tamari
  soy sauce

2 tablespoons dry sherry

freshly ground black pepper,
  to taste

In a large nonstick skillet, melt butter over medium-high heat. When butter is hot and bubbly, add scallions and mushrooms and sauté until mushrooms are tender, about 5 minutes. Stir in soy sauce, sherry and black pepper.

Sesame Broccoli

Makes 6 side-dish servings • Each serving: 3 grams protein • trace carbohydrate

2 teaspoons raw sesame seeds,
  for garnish

2 bunches broccoli, cut into
  bite-size florets

1 tablespoon pure-pressed
  sesame oil

1 tablespoon rice wine vinegar

2 teaspoons low-sodium tamari
  soy sauce

freshly ground black pepper,
  to taste

Put sesame seeds in an ungreased skillet over medium-high heat. Stir seeds or shake pan almost constantly until seeds are evenly browned and toasted and begin to pop. Remove from pan immediately and set aside.

In a large saucepan, bring 2 cups water to a boil. Add broccoli florets and cook until barely tender, about 5 to 7 minutes. Drain and set aside.

In a small bowl, using a fork, mix sesame oil, rice wine vinegar, soy sauce and black pepper. Toss gently with steamed broccoli. Taste, and adjust seasonings. Sprinkle with sesame seeds before serving.

Sun-Dried Tomato Cooked Spinach

Makes 4 side-dish servings • Each serving: 3 grams protein • 7 grams carbohydrate

*2 bunches spinach equal to about
2 cups cooked spinach, well
drained and chopped; or
16 ounces packaged frozen
spinach, thawed, drained
and chopped*

*½ cup Sun-Dried Tomato Pesto
(see recipe, page 295), or
store-bought*

¼ cup all-dairy heavy cream

Wash spinach well, removing stems. With water still clinging to leaves, place in a medium saucepan with a tight-fitting lid. Turn heat to medium-high and steam until leaves are wilted, about 2 to 3 minutes. Drain in a colander, pressing out all liquid with the back of a wooden spoon. Chop fine and set aside.

In a food processor, blend cooked and drained spinach with tomato pesto and cream until smooth. Taste, and adjust seasonings.

Transfer to a small saucepan and gently heat through. *Do not boil.*

Vegetable Stir-Fry

Makes 4 side-dish servings • Each serving: 3 grams protein • 2 grams carbohydrate

2 tablespoons pure-pressed
peanut oil

2 teaspoons peeled and finely
minced fresh ginger

2 minced garlic cloves

1 cup thinly slivered carrots

1 cup thinly slivered zucchini

1 thinly sliced green or red bell
pepper

2 cups thinly sliced brown or
white mushrooms

1 tablespoon low-sodium tamari
soy sauce

½ cup vegetable stock (see recipe,
page 100), or low-sodium
canned, or water

2 teaspoons pure-pressed sesame
oil

1 tablespoon chopped scallions

In a wok or a large nonstick skillet, heat oil over medium-high heat. When oil is hot, add ginger and garlic and stir-fry, about 30 seconds. Add carrots, zucchini and bell pepper and stir-fry 2 minutes. Add mushrooms and stir-fry 2 more minutes.

Sprinkle with soy sauce and stir-fry until well blended. Add stock or water and turn heat to high. Cover and cook about 2 minutes, or until vegetables are tender.

Sprinkle with sesame oil and chopped scallions.

Zucchini Eggplant Tomato Trio

Makes 4 side-dish servings • Each serving: 4 grams protein • 2 grams carbohydrate

2 tablespoons pure-pressed extra virgin olive oil

2 medium thinly sliced red onions

2 minced garlic cloves

4 ripe medium tomatoes

4 medium zucchini

3 small Japanese eggplants (peeled, if desired)

¼ cup pure-pressed extra virgin olive oil

freshly ground black pepper, to taste

1 tablespoon chopped fresh thyme, or 2 teaspoons dried thyme

2 tablespoons grated Parmesan cheese

Preheat oven to 350°. In a large nonstick skillet, heat oil over medium-high heat. When oil is hot, add onion and garlic, and sauté until softened, about 5 minutes. Spread onion in bottom of an 8-inch-square baking dish.

Slice tomatoes, zucchini and eggplant into thin ¼-inch slices. On top of onion, make a row of sliced zucchini down the length of baking pan. Next, make a row of eggplant, overlapping zucchini about halfway. Next, make a row of tomato slices, overlapping eggplant row by half. Continue making rows until all vegetables are used.

Drizzle olive oil over vegetables. Sprinkle with black pepper and thyme. Bake until vegetables are tender, about 30 minutes. Increase oven temperature to 475°. Sprinkle with grated Parmesan cheese and cook 5 minutes, until top is lightly browned.

Zucchini with Basil, Parmesan Cheese and Toasted Almonds

Makes 4 side-dish servings • Each serving: 2 grams protein • trace carbohydrate

2 tablespoons raw sliced
  almonds, for garnish

4 medium zucchini

2 tablespoons pure-pressed extra
  virgin olive oil

1 minced garlic clove

freshly ground black pepper,
  to taste

1 tablespoon slivered fresh basil,
  or 1 teaspoon dried basil

2 tablespoons grated Parmesan
  cheese

Put almonds in an ungreased skillet over medium-high heat. Stir or shake pan almost constantly, until almonds are evenly browned and toasted. Remove from pan immediately and set aside.

Trim ends of zucchini and cut lengthwise into ¼-inch-thick long slices. Cut slices into 1-inch squares.

In a large nonstick skillet, heat oil over medium-high heat. When oil is hot, add garlic and zucchini and sauté until zucchini is tender, about 5 to 7 minutes. Stir frequently. Remove from heat, add black pepper, basil and Parmesan cheese. Taste, and adjust seasonings.

Transfer to a serving bowl and sprinkle with sliced almonds.

Starchy Vegetable Side Dishes

Garlic Mashed Potatoes

Makes 6 side-dish servings • Each serving: 3 grams protein • 26 grams carbohydrate

1 bulb garlic

*1½ pounds russet potatoes
(peeled, if desired)*

*⅓ cup all-dairy heavy cream,
heated to simmering*

*3 tablespoons melted unsalted
butter*

*freshly ground black pepper,
to taste*

Preheat oven to 450°. With a sharp knife, slice off the top ½ inch of the garlic bulb and discard or save for another use. Drizzle the bulb with olive oil and black pepper. In a small baking dish, bake garlic until cloves are browned and pop out of their skins, about 15 to 20 minutes. Set aside. When cool, squeeze cloves out of skins and mince.

Cook potatoes in boiling water until fork-tender, about 15 to 20 minutes. Drain and return to pot. Mash with a fork or potato masher, adding heated cream, butter and roasted garlic. Season to taste with black pepper.

Jitka Gunaratna's Potato Pancakes

Makes 4 side-dish servings • Each serving: 5 grams protein • 26 grams carbohydrate

2 large russet baking potatoes

1 egg

2 to 3 minced garlic cloves

1 teaspoon dried marjoram

freshly ground black pepper, to taste

3 tablespoons unsalted butter

Peel and grate potatoes. Place grated potatoes in a sieve for 10 minutes to drain into a bowl. Set drained water aside to allow starch to settle to bottom of bowl.

In medium bowl, beat egg with a fork. Add drained potatoes, garlic, marjoram and black pepper. Mix well. Drain potato water from bowl and discard. Mix remaining starch, from bottom of the bowl, into potato mixture.

In a large nonstick skillet, melt butter. When butter is hot and bubbly, spoon dollops of batter into pan. Form pancakes by flattening slightly with the back of a spoon. Cook until golden brown on bottom before turning. Drain on paper towels.

Oven-Roasted Sweet Potatoes

Makes 6 side-dish servings • Each serving: 1 gram protein • 14 grams carbohydrate

1½ pounds sweet potatoes

3 tablespoons pure-pressed extra virgin olive oil

freshly ground black pepper, to taste

Preheat oven to 450°. Peel sweet potatoes and cut into 1½-inch chunks. Toss with olive oil and black pepper. Spread in a single layer on a greased baking sheet. Roast about 20 to 30 minutes, turning occasionally, until evenly browned and tender.

Potato Gratin

Makes 6 side-dish servings • Each serving: 6 grams protein • 42 grams carbohydrate

2 tablespoons unsalted butter

2 minced garlic cloves

1 tablespoon flour

1 cup all-dairy heavy cream,
  heated to simmering

2¼ pounds russet potatoes
  (peeled, if desired) cut into
  ¼-inch-thick rounds

freshly ground black pepper,
  to taste

1 tablespoon melted unsalted
  butter

¼ cup fresh or dried whole-grain
  bread crumbs

¼ cup grated Parmesan cheese

Preheat oven to 350°. In a small nonstick skillet, melt 2 tablespoons butter over medium-high heat. When butter is hot and bubbly, add garlic and stir until softened, about 30 seconds. Add flour and cook 3 minutes, stirring constantly. Stir in heated cream and bring to a simmer, stirring occasionally, cooking until thickened, about 1 to 2 minutes. *Do not boil.*

Butter an oven-proof 11-inch casserole or similar size dish. Arrange potatoes in overlapping layers. Season to taste with black pepper. Pour cream mixture over top.

Bake 1 hour or longer, until potatoes are tender. Sprinkle with melted butter, bread crumbs and Parmesan cheese and place briefly under broiler until lightly browned.

Puréed Acorn Squash

Makes 4 side-dish servings • Each serving: 12 grams protein • 14 grams carbohydrate

2 acorn squash, cut in half and
  seeded

2 tablespoons unsalted butter

freshly ground black pepper,
  to taste

Preheat oven to 450°. Place squash, cavity-side up, in a baking pan. Add 1 inch of water to pan to prevent burning. Dot ½ tablespoon of butter into each squash cavity. Roast in oven, uncovered, until squash is tender and lightly browned, about 30 to 40 minutes.

Scoop out squash pulp and discard skin. In a blender or food processor, purée pulp until smooth. Season to taste with black pepper.

Roasted Potatoes with Garlic and Cheese

Makes 6 side-dish servings • Each serving: 7 grams protein • 20 grams carbohydrate

2 pounds small, red potatoes
  (peeled, if desired)

1½ tablespoons pure-pressed
  extra virgin olive oil

freshly ground black pepper,
  to taste

10 whole peeled garlic cloves,
  mixed with 1 teaspoon pure-
  pressed extra virgin olive oil

½ cup crumbled feta or
  Gorgonzola cheese

2 tablespoons minced fresh
  parsley

Preheat oven to 475°. Slice potatoes into quarters. In a large bowl, toss with olive oil and black pepper.

Spread potatoes on a lightly greased baking sheet and roast 30 minutes, turning occasionally. Add whole garlic cloves the last 15 minutes. Remove from oven and toss gently with feta or Gorgonzola cheese and minced parsley.

Stir-Fried Red Potatoes and Cabbage

Makes 6 side-dish servings • Each serving: 3 grams protein • 13 grams carbohydrate

2 tablespoons pure-pressed extra
  virgin olive oil

1 tablespoon unsalted butter

4 medium red potatoes
  (peeled, if desired) diced into
  ½-inch cubes

2 teaspoons peeled and finely
  minced fresh ginger

1 teaspoon ground cumin

¼ teaspoon red-pepper flakes

1 pound finely sliced Napa or
  Savoy cabbage

freshly ground black pepper,
  to taste

In a large nonstick skillet, heat oil and butter over medium-high heat. When hot, add diced potatoes, ginger, cumin and red-pepper flakes. Sauté until potatoes are evenly browned and tender, about 15 minutes. Add cabbage and stir constantly, until tender and bright green, about 5 minutes. Season to taste with black pepper.

Stuffed Baked Potatoes

Makes 8 side-dish servings • Each side-dish serving: 9 grams protein • 35 grams carbohydrate

4 large baking potatoes

2 tablespoons pure-pressed extra virgin olive oil

1 small diced onion

1 cup chopped brown or white mushrooms

¼ cup pesto (see Pestos, starting on page 293), or store-bought

½ cup crumbled feta cheese

freshly ground black pepper, to taste

paprika, for garnish

Preheat oven to 425°. Scrub potatoes and prick with a knife in several places. Bake directly on oven rack 1 hour or until soft. Cut potatoes in half lengthwise and scoop out insides, leaving a ¼-inch-thick shell.

In a medium nonstick skillet, heat oil over medium-high heat. When oil is hot, add onion and mushrooms and sauté until softened and all mushroom liquid has been absorbed, about 6 to 8 minutes. In a large bowl, combine scooped-out potato filling, onion and mushrooms, pesto, crumbled feta cheese and black pepper.

Stuff mixture back into potato shells, mounding on top. Place on a baking sheet. Reduce oven temperature to 350° and bake until heated through, about 30 minutes. Sprinkle tops of potatoes with paprika before serving.

Chutney,
Compound Butters,
Mayonnaise, Pestos,
Salsas and Sauces

Chutney

Compound Butters

Mayonnaise

Pestos

Salsas

Sauces

Chutney

Apricot and Raisin Chutney

Makes about 1 cup • 1 tablespoon: 1 gram protein • 7 grams carbohydrate

Serve with Indian curries.

½ cup raisins

½ cup dried apricots

½ cup boiling water

2 tablespoons fresh lime juice

dash cayenne pepper

In a small bowl, soak raisins and apricots in boiling water for 15 minutes. Transfer to a blender or food processor and add lime juice and cayenne pepper. Process until well blended and smooth. Taste, and adjust seasonings. Cover and refrigerate.

Compound Butters

To prepare compound butter, let 1 stick of butter soften at room temperature. Mix in fresh herbs and seasonings. Scoop blended butter onto center of a piece of plastic wrap or waxed paper. Roll into a 6-inch log, sealing edges. Refrigerate until firm. Cut off pats of butter as needed. (The logs may also be frozen.) To serve, melt a pat of compound butter on any hot dish.

Caper Butter

Makes about ½ cup • 1 tablespoon: trace protein • trace carbohydrate

1 stick unsalted butter

2 tablespoons rinsed and drained chopped capers

2 tablespoons chopped fresh tarragon, or 2 teaspoons dried tarragon

freshly ground black pepper, to taste

Curry Butter

Makes about ½ cup • 1 tablespoon: trace protein • trace carbohydrate

1 stick unsalted butter

1 teaspoon curry powder

1 teaspoon minced fresh cilantro

1 teaspoon minced scallions

freshly ground black pepper, to taste

Fresh Basil Butter

Makes about ½ cup • 1 tablespoon: trace protein • trace carbohydrate

1 stick unsalted butter

1 tablespoon fresh lemon juice

2 tablespoons slivered fresh basil,
   or 2 teaspoons dried basil

freshly ground black pepper,
   to taste

Fresh Lemon Butter

Makes about ½ cup • 1 tablespoon: trace protein • trace carbohydrate

1 stick unsalted butter

1 tablespoon fresh lemon juice

1 teaspoon grated lemon zest

1 tablespoon minced fresh parsley

freshly ground black pepper,
   to taste

Garlic Cilantro Lime Butter

Makes about ½ cup • 1 tablespoon: trace protein • trace carbohydrate

1 stick unsalted butter

2 tablespoons chopped fresh
   cilantro

2 teaspoons fresh lime juice

2 minced garlic cloves

freshly ground black pepper,
   to taste

Mayonnaise

Aioli (Garlic Mayonnaise)

Makes about 1¼ cups • 1 tablespoon: trace protein • trace carbohydrate

Use as a dip for vegetables, or as a sandwich spread.

1 egg yolk*

3 minced garlic cloves

*freshly ground black pepper,
   to taste*

½ cup pure-pressed canola oil

*½ cup pure-pressed extra virgin
   olive oil*

*2 to 3 teaspoons fresh lemon
   juice, to taste*

In a blender or food processor, blend egg yolk, garlic and black pepper on high until smooth. With motor running, gradually drizzle in oils until creamy and thickened. Add lemon juice and blend well. Store covered in refrigerator.

Creamy Mayonnaise

Makes about 1 cup • 1 tablespoon: trace protein • trace carbohydrate

Delicious with steamed vegetables, or as a sandwich spread.

1 egg yolk*

2 tablespoons fresh lemon juice

1 tablespoon Dijon mustard

*freshly ground black pepper,
   to taste*

¾ cup pure-pressed canola oil

In a blender or food processor, blend egg yolk, lemon juice, mustard and black pepper until smooth. With motor running, gradually pour in oil until creamy and thickened. Store covered in refrigerator.

*If you are concerned about using raw eggs, choose an alternate recipe.

Curried Mayonnaise

Makes about 1¼ cups • 1 tablespoon: trace protein • trace carbohydrate

Serve with steamed artichokes or asparagus, or as a sandwich spread.

1 egg yolk*

2 tablespoons fresh lime juice

1 tablespoon Dijon mustard

1 tablespoon curry powder

2 teaspoons grated lime zest

*freshly ground black pepper,
  to taste*

*½ cup pure-pressed extra virgin
  olive oil*

½ cup pure-pressed canola oil

In a blender or food processor, blend egg yolk, lime juice, mustard, curry powder, lime zest and black pepper until smooth. With motor running, gradually drizzle in oils until creamy and thickened. Store covered in refrigerator.

———————

*If you are concerned about using raw eggs, choose an alternate recipe.

Garlic Caper Mayonnaise

Makes about 1¼ cups • 1 tablespoon: trace protein • trace carbohydrate

Delicious as a dip for steamed artichokes or raw vegetables.

1 egg yolk*

2 tablespoons fresh lemon juice

1 minced garlic clove

1 tablespoon drained and rinsed
capers

freshly ground black pepper,
to taste

dash cayenne pepper

½ cup pure-pressed extra virgin
olive oil

½ cup pure-pressed canola oil

2 tablespoons minced fresh
parsley

In a blender or food processor, blend egg yolk, lemon juice, garlic, capers, black pepper and cayenne pepper until smooth. With motor running, gradually add oils until creamy and thickened. Stir in parsley. Store covered in refrigerator.

———————

*If you are concerned about using raw eggs, choose an alternate recipe.

Pestos

Asian Pesto

Makes about 1 cup • 2 tablespoons: 1 gram protein • 1 gram carbohydrate

Serve with grilled vegetables or baked tofu.

1 cup loosely packed fresh mint leaves

1 cup loosely packed fresh cilantro

1 cup loosely packed fresh basil leaves

¼ cup pure-pressed extra virgin olive oil

¼ cup chopped raw walnuts

2 tablespoons fresh lime juice

2 minced garlic cloves

freshly ground black pepper, to taste

In a blender or food processor, purée all ingredients. Taste, and adjust seasonings. Store covered in refrigerator.

Basil Pesto

Makes about ¾ cup • 2 tablespoons: 6 grams protein • 2 grams carbohydrate

Serve with omelets, grilled vegetables, baked potatoes, or as a sandwich spread.

2 cups packed fresh basil leaves

2 chopped garlic cloves

3 tablespoons raw pine nuts or raw walnuts

⅓ cup grated Parmesan cheese

⅓ cup pure-pressed extra virgin olive oil

freshly ground black pepper, to taste

dash cayenne pepper

In a blender or food processor, purée all ingredients. Taste, and adjust seasonings. Store covered in refrigerator.

Cilantro Pesto

Makes about 1 cup • 2 tablespoons: 3 grams protein • 2 grams carbohydrate

Serve with grilled vegetables or cheese quesadillas.

2 bunches cilantro, coarsely chopped with stems removed

2 tablespoons fresh lime juice

½ cup roasted and chopped pumpkin seeds

½ cup grated Parmesan cheese

6 minced garlic cloves

½ cup pure-pressed extra virgin olive oil

freshly ground black pepper, to taste

In a blender or food processor, purée all ingredients. Taste, and adjust seasonings. Store covered in refrigerator.

Sun-Dried Tomato Pesto

Makes about 1 cup • 2 tablespoons: 3 grams protein • 7 grams carbohydrate

Serve with grilled vegetables, grilled-cheese sandwiches or baked potatoes.

1 cup sun-dried tomatoes in olive oil

2 tablespoons slivered fresh basil, or 1 teaspoon dried basil

¼ cup grated Parmesan cheese

1 minced garlic clove

⅛ teaspoon red-pepper flakes

In a food processor, purée tomatoes with their oil, basil, Parmesan cheese, garlic and red-pepper flakes. Taste, and adjust seasonings. Store covered in refrigerator.

Salsas

Fresh Mexican Salsa

Makes about 2¾ cups • Each ¼ cup serving: trace protein • 2 grams carbohydrate

Serve with grilled vegetables, cheese quesadillas or enchiladas.

2 cups diced ripe tomatoes

2 minced garlic cloves

2 tablespoons diced red onion

2 tablespoons chopped scallions

2 tablespoons minced fresh cilantro

1 small diced fresh jalapeño pepper; or 1 to 2 tablespoons canned diced green chilies, to taste [wear rubber gloves to prepare fresh jalapeño pepper]

2 tablespoons pure-pressed extra virgin olive oil

1 to 2 tablespoons fresh lemon or lime juice, to taste

1 teaspoon dried oregano

freshly ground black pepper, to taste

In a medium bowl, combine all ingredients. Taste, and adjust seasonings. Chill before serving.

Fresh Papaya or Mango Salsa

Makes about 3 cups • Each ¼ cup serving Papaya Salsa: trace protein • 2 grams carbohydrate
Each ¼ cup serving Mango Salsa: trace protein • 6 grams carbohydrate

Serve with grilled vegetables, cheese quesadillas or enchiladas.

1 small minced red onion

1 small minced fresh jalapeño pepper; or 1 to 2 tablespoons canned diced green chilies, to taste [wear rubber gloves to prepare fresh jalapeño pepper]

½ cup diced red bell pepper

2 minced garlic cloves

2 cups diced papaya, or 2 cups diced mango

*1 seeded and diced ripe medium tomato**

2 tablespoons minced fresh cilantro

2 tablespoons minced scallions

2 tablespoons fresh lime juice

1 tablespoon pure-pressed extra virgin olive oil

freshly ground black pepper, to taste

In a medium bowl, combine all ingredients and mix well. Taste, and adjust seasonings. Refrigerate 1 hour before serving.

---

* To seed tomatoes: Cut tomatoes in half and gently squeeze. Scoop out seeds and pulp with a small spoon or your fingers.

Fresh Salsa Verde

Makes about 2 cups • 2 tablespoons: trace protein • trace carbohydrate

Serve with grilled vegetables, baked tofu or cheese quesadillas.

½ cup chopped fresh cilantro

½ cup slivered fresh basil

½ cup chopped fresh parsley

½ cup chopped scallions

2 minced garlic cloves

⅓ cup balsamic vinegar

freshly ground black pepper, to taste

1 cup pure-pressed extra virgin olive oil

In a food processor, blend all ingredients except olive oil. With motor running, slowly drizzle in olive oil until well blended. Taste, and adjust seasonings. Store covered in refrigerator.

Fresh Thai Salsa

Makes about 2½ cups • Each ¼ cup serving: trace protein • trace carbohydrate

Serve with roasted vegetables, grilled tofu or cheese quesadillas.

2 tablespoons chopped scallions

⅓ cup fresh lime juice

2 tablespoons minced fresh cilantro

2 minced garlic cloves

2 tablespoons slivered fresh basil

1 tablespoon minced fresh mint

4 seeded and diced ripe medium
  tomatoes*

¼ cup diced red onion

2 teaspoons peeled and finely
  minced fresh ginger

1 tablespoon balsamic vinegar

½ cup pure-pressed extra virgin
  olive oil

freshly ground black pepper,
  to taste

In a medium bowl, combine all ingredients. Mix well. Taste, and adjust seasonings. Store covered in refrigerator.

To seed tomatoes: Cut tomatoes in half and gently squeeze. Scoop out seeds with a small spoon or your fingers.

Sauces

Basic Tomato Sauce

Makes about 5 cups • Each ½ cup serving: 1 gram protein • 5 grams carbohydrate

Serve with tofu "meatballs," roasted eggplant and steamed grains.

2 tablespoons pure-pressed extra
  virgin olive oil

1 medium chopped onion

4 minced garlic cloves

28 ounces canned crushed
  tomatoes, (reserve liquid)

¼ cup tomato paste

½ cup red wine

1 bay leaf

2 teaspoons dried oregano

¼ teaspoon red-pepper flakes

½ cup slivered fresh basil, or
  2 teaspoons dried basil

¼ cup finely chopped fresh
  parsley

freshly ground black pepper,
  to taste

In a large saucepan, heat oil over medium-high heat. When oil is hot, add onion and garlic and sauté over medium heat until softened, about 5 minutes. Add tomatoes and their liquid, tomato paste, red wine, bay leaf, oregano, red-pepper flakes, basil, parsley and black pepper. Stir well. Bring to a boil. Reduce heat and simmer 30 minutes, stirring occasionally. Taste, and adjust seasonings.

Cilantro Lime Sauce

Makes about 1 cup • 2 tablespoons: trace protein • trace carbohydrate

Serve with steamed grains, grilled tofu or steamed vegetables.

1 stick unsalted butter

½ cup chopped red onion

2 minced garlic cloves

3 tablespoons fresh lime juice

2 teaspoons grated lime zest

dash hot-pepper sauce

2 tablespoons chopped fresh cilantro

freshly ground black pepper, to taste

In a medium nonstick skillet, melt butter over medium-high heat. When butter is hot and bubbly, add onion and garlic and cook until softened, about 5 minutes. Add lime juice, zest, hot-pepper sauce, cilantro and black pepper. Simmer 5 minutes over medium-low heat. Transfer to a blender or food processor and blend until smooth. Taste, and adjust seasonings.

Classic Blender Hollandaise Sauce

Makes about 1 cup • Each ¼ cup serving: 2½ grams protein • trace carbohydrate

Serve with poached eggs and steamed vegetables.

3 egg yolks*

2 tablespoons fresh lemon juice

dash cayenne pepper

4 ounces (1 stick) unsalted butter,
melted and bubbling hot

In a blender, combine egg yolks, lemon juice and cayenne pepper, on high for 3 seconds. Remove lid and, with motor running, slowly pour hot butter in a steady stream over eggs. When butter is all poured in, blend an additional 5 seconds. Taste, and adjust seasonings. Serve immediately, or keep sauce warm by placing blender in a bowl of warm water.

———————

*If you are concerned about using raw eggs, choose an alternate recipe.

Coconut Curry Sauce

Makes about 1½ cups • Each ¼ cup serving: 2 grams protein • trace carbohydrate

Serve with baked tofu, grilled vegetables or steamed rice.

1 tablespoon unsalted butter	½ cup coconut milk
1½ tablespoons curry powder	1 tablespoon shredded
2 minced garlic cloves	unsweetened coconut
2 teaspoons peeled and finely minced fresh ginger	1 tablespoon minced fresh cilantro
¼ teaspoon ground cardamom	2 teaspoons minced fresh mint
1 teaspoon mustard seeds	freshly ground black pepper, to taste
¾ cup all-dairy heavy cream	

In a medium saucepan, melt butter over medium-high heat. When butter is hot and bubbly, add curry powder, garlic, ginger, cardamom and mustard seeds. Reduce heat to medium and sauté 2 to 3 minutes, until mustard seeds begin to pop.

Add cream, coconut milk, coconut, cilantro, mint and black pepper. Mix well with a wooden spoon. Simmer gently 5 minutes, stirring until thickened and well mixed. Taste, and adjust seasonings.

Cooling Mint Sauce

Makes about 1½ cups • Each ¼ cup serving: 2 grams protein • 2 grams carbohydrate

Serve with Indian main-course curries.

1 cup whole plain yogurt

1 teaspoon grated lime zest

1 tablespoon finely chopped fresh mint

½ cup peeled, seeded and diced cucumber

In a small bowl, using a fork or wooden spoon, combine yogurt, lime zest, mint and cucumber until well blended. Store covered in refrigerator.

Enchilada Sauce

Makes about 3 cups • Each ½ cup serving: 2 grams protein • 6 grams carbohydrate

Serve with Cheesy Enchiladas or Huevos Rancheros.

*2 tablespoons pure-pressed
  extra virgin olive oil*

1 large diced onion

3 minced garlic cloves

*1 small minced fresh jalapeño
  pepper; or 1 to 2 tablespoons
  canned green chilies, to taste
  [wear rubber gloves to
  prepare fresh jalapeño pepper]*

2 teaspoons ground cumin

2 teaspoons dried oregano

2 teaspoons chili powder

*freshly ground black pepper,
  to taste*

*28 ounces canned tomatoes,
  puréed, (reserve liquid)*

*1 to 2 tablespoons fresh lime
  juice, to taste*

*1 tablespoon minced fresh
  cilantro*

In a large saucepan, heat oil over medium-high heat. When oil is hot, add onion, garlic, jalapeño pepper, cumin, oregano, chili powder and black pepper. Sauté until onion is softened, about 5 minutes. Add tomatoes and their liquid, mix well and bring to a boil. Reduce heat to low, and simmer uncovered 15 to 20 minutes. Add lime juice and minced cilantro. Taste, and adjust seasonings.

Herbed Caper Butter

Makes about ½ cup • 1 tablespoon: 1 gram protein • trace carbohydrate

Serve with baked potatoes, steamed vegetables or grains.

4 tablespoons unsalted butter

1 tablespoon drained and rinsed capers

1 tablespoon fresh lemon juice

1 teaspoon dried oregano

freshly ground black pepper, to taste

In a small saucepan, melt butter over low heat. When butter is melted, add remaining ingredients. Heat through. Taste, and adjust seasonings. Serve warm.

Mustard Sauce

Makes about 1½ cups • Each ¼ cup serving: 1 gram protein • trace carbohydrate

Delicious with grilled vegetables or baked tofu.

2 egg yolks*

2 teaspoons red wine vinegar

dash white pepper

1 tablespoon fresh lemon juice

1 minced garlic clove

3 tablespoons Dijon mustard

1 cup pure-pressed canola oil

In a blender or food processor, blend all ingredients except oil. With motor running, drizzle in oil until sauce is smooth. Taste, and adjust seasonings. Store covered in refrigerator.

———————

*If you are concerned about using raw eggs, choose an alternate recipe.

Quick Blender Béarnaise Sauce

Makes about 1½ cups • Each ¼ cup serving: 2 grams protein • trace carbohydrate

Delicious with omelets and steamed vegetables.

2 tablespoons white wine

1 tablespoon tarragon vinegar

1 tablespoon chopped fresh
tarragon

1 tablespoon chopped shallots

freshly ground black pepper,
to taste

3 egg yolks*

2 tablespoons fresh lemon juice

dash cayenne pepper

½ cup melted, bubbly hot
unsalted butter

In a small saucepan, combine wine, vinegar, tarragon, shallots and black pepper. Bring to a boil and cook until reduced by half.

In a blender, combine egg yolks with lemon juice and cayenne pepper, on high. With motor running, gradually drizzle in hot melted butter. Add wine/herb mixture and blend on high until creamy and thickened. Taste, and adjust seasonings.

———————

*If you are concerned about using raw eggs, choose an alternate recipe.

Shitake Mushroom Gravy

Makes about 2¼ cups • Each 2 tablespoon serving: trace protein • trace carbohydrate

1 ounce dried shitake mushrooms

2 tablespoons unsalted butter

1 medium chopped onion

1 minced garlic clove

2 tablespoons dry sherry

1 teaspoon paprika

1 tablespoon low-sodium tamari soy sauce

4 tablespoons butter

3 tablespoons flour

2 cups reserved shitake mushroom soaking liquid or vegetable stock (see recipe, page 100), heated

2 tablespoons chopped fresh parsley

freshly ground black pepper, to taste

Cover shitake mushrooms with 3 cups hot water and let stand for about 20 minutes. Remove from water, strain liquid and set aside. Cut coarse stem end off of mushrooms and discard. Slice mushroom caps into ¼-inch strips.

In a large skillet, melt 2 tablespoons butter over medium-high heat. When butter is hot and bubbly, add onions, garlic and mushrooms. Sauté 8 minutes, stirring frequently.

Add sherry, paprika and soy sauce and cook 1 minute before transferring mushroom mixture to a bowl.

Melt 4 tablespoons butter in pan over medium-high heat. When butter is hot and bubbly, add flour and whisk, stirring and cooking for 5 minutes.

Meanwhile, heat reserved mushroom liquid or stock to almost boiling. Slowly add hot mushroom liquid or stock to butter and flour mixture. Cook until thickened, stirring frequently, about 5 minutes.

Stir in sautéed mushroom mixture, parsley and black pepper. Taste, and adjust seasonings. Serve as is or blend in food processor or blender until smooth.

Spicy Peanut Sauce

Makes about 1¼ cups • Each ¼ cup serving: 4 grams protein • 4 grams carbohydrate

Serve with grilled vegetables, baked tofu or steamed brown rice.

5 chopped garlic cloves

2 tablespoons peeled and finely minced fresh ginger

½ cup chopped fresh cilantro

2 tablespoons pure-pressed sesame oil

1 tablespoon hot chili oil

½ cup organic peanut butter (no honey or sugar added)

¼ cup low-sodium tamari soy sauce

2 tablespoons fresh lime juice

1 tablespoon rice wine vinegar

dash cayenne pepper

hot water if needed to thin

In a food processor, blend garlic, ginger and cilantro. Add oils, peanut butter, soy sauce, lime juice, vinegar and cayenne pepper and blend until smooth and creamy, scraping down sides of bowl. Add hot water for a thinner consistency. Taste, and adjust seasonings, adding more soy sauce or lime juice, if desired.

Index

A

accelerated metabolic aging, 2, 7, 9
Acorn Squash, Puréed, 281
African Quinoa Soup with Vegetables,
 95
Aioli (Garlic Mayonnaise)
 in Mushroom Tofu Burger, 197
 recipe, 290
alcohol tips, 10
"all-dairy" tips, 9
almonds
 in Brown Rice with Mushrooms, 244
 in Chutney Dip, 77
 Curried Almond Dressing, 127
 in Green Onion and Lime Rice, 246
 in Mushroom Kasha Pilaf, 231
 in Spicy Mixed Nuts, 73
 in Spinach Rice Pilaf, 248
 in Zucchini with Basil and Parmesan
  Cheese, 274
Annette Matrisciano's Cheesy Eggs, 19
Anytime Soup, 101
appetizers and snacks, 65–74
 Artichokes with Hollandaise Sauce,
  65
 Asparagus Spears in Garlic
  Vinaigrette, 66
 Cheesy Quesadillas, 67
 Curried Deviled Eggs, 68
 Mushrooms, Marinated, 69
 Pecan Cheese Ball, 70
 Salad Stix, 71

Sesame Baked Mushrooms, 72
Spicy Mixed Nuts, 73
Spinach-and-Cheese-Stuffed
 Mushrooms, 74
See also dips; spreads
apples, in Curried Spinach Salad with
 Almond Dressing, 127
Apricot and Raisin Chutney
 in Chutney Dip, 77
 in Curried Tofu Scramble, 53
 recipe, 287
artichokes
 in Breakfast Strata, 20
 Cheese Dip, Famous Hot, 79
 Creamy Chowder, 106
 in Crustless Quiche, with Variations,
  23
 in Greek-Salad-Filled Pita Breads,
  188
 with Hollandaise Sauce, 65
 and Mushroom Frittata, 33
 and Mushroom Salad, 135
 in Salad Stix, 71
 and Spinach with Kalamata Olives,
  204
Asian
 Citrus Dressing, 151
 Mint Pesto, 167
 Mint Pesto Tofu Kabobs, 167
 Pesto, 293
 Scramble, 47

nonstarchy vegetable side dishes *(continued)*
Creamed Spinach with Mushrooms, 258
Crustless Zucchini Quiche, 259
Curried Cauliflower, 260
Eggplant, Broiled, 257
Green Beans in Peanut Sauce, 261
Green Beans with Sesame Mayonnaise, 262
Indonesian Asparagus, 263
Italian Cauliflower, 264
Mushrooms, Sautéed, 269
Pepper (Roasted) Medley, 267
Piperade (Bell Pepper and Tomato Stew), 265
Ratatouille, 266
Sesame Broccoli, 270
Spinach (Baked) and Feta-Filled Tomatoes, 255
Squash, Sautéed Mixed, with Cumin and Chili Powder, 268
Sun-Dried Tomato Cooked Spinach, 271
Vegetable Stir-Fry, 272
Zucchini Eggplant Tomato Trio, 273
Zucchini with Basil, Parmesan Cheese and Toasted Almonds, 274
nonstarchy vegetables nutrient group, 3, 7, 8
nutrition, balanced, 3–4, 7–8, 95
nutritional analysis of recipes, 8
nuts
Spicy Mixed, 73
See also almonds; cashew nuts; peanuts; pecans; pine nuts; pistachio nuts; walnuts

O

Oatmeal with Butter and Cream, 28
oils, pure-pressed, 10
olives. *See* green olives; Kalamata olives
omelets, 38–45
Cream Cheese and Avocado Omelet, 38
Curried Tofu Omelet, 39
Greek Omelet, 40

Mushroom and Gorgonzola Omelet with Walnuts, 41
Soy Sausage and Cheese Omelet, 42
Spinach and Brie Omelet, 43
Sun-Dried Tomato and Chèvre (Goat Cheese) Omelet, 44
Western Omelet, 45
See also eggs, scrambled; frittatas; pestos; sauces
onions
in Barley and Mushroom Casserole, 227
and Beet Salad, 119
in Black Bean and Goat Cheese Enchiladas, 170–71
in Black Bean Chili, 172
in Broccoli and Mushroom Sauce, 191
in Brown Rice Pilaf, 243
in California Coleslaw, 120
in Caponata Salad, 121
in Cauliflower Potato Soup, 103
and Cheese, Soy Sausage Frittata, 35
in Cheesy Enchiladas, 176
in Cilantro Lime Sauce, 301
in Coconut Cashew Nut Curry, 179
in Creamed Spinach with Mushrooms, 258
in Creamy Artichoke Chowder, 106
in Creamy Broccoli Soup, 107
in Creamy Roasted Eggplant Soup, 108
in Creamy Spinach Soup, 109
in Creamy Tomato Soup, 110
in Crustless Zucchini Quiche, 259
in Curried Cauliflower, 260
in Curried Millet, 236
in Enchilada Sauce, 305
in Feta Cheese and Mushroom Quesadillas, 187
French (Very) Onion Soup, 114
in Garbanzo Bean Salad, 128
in Greek Rice, 245
in Greek Salad, 129
in Greek-Salad-Filled Pita Breads, 188

in Pear and Gorgonzola Winter
Salad, 136
Red Cabbage with Walnuts Salad,
138
in Ricotta-Stuffed Bell Peppers, 202
in Spinach (Baked) and Feta-Filled
Tomatoes, 255
water chestnuts, in Szechwan Tofu with
Green Beans, Mushrooms and
Peanuts, 207–8
Western Omelet, 45
wheat berries, in Brown Rice Pilaf, 243
wild rice, in Brown Rice Pilaf, 243
Winter Vinaigrette, 136

Y
yogurt
in Curried Cauliflower, 260
in Mint Sauce, Cooling, 304
Peanut Butter Smoothie with Yogurt
and Banana, 60
Peanut Butter Smoothie with Yogurt
and Dates, 61
Smoothie with Cottage Cheese and
Strawberries, 61
in Tahini Sauce, 186
in Tandoori-Style Tofu, 210
in Thousand Island Dressing, 164
tips, 10

Z
zucchini
in African Quinoa Soup with
Vegetables, 95
with Basil, Parmesan Cheese and
Toasted Almonds, 274
and Corn Medley, 223
Crustless Zucchini Quiche, 259
in Egg Foo Yung with Rice Crust,
181–82
and Eggplant Tomato Trio, 273
in Italian Mixed Vegetable Soup, 111
in Middle Eastern Lentils with
Vegetables, 234
in Moroccan Curried Lentil Soup, 97
in Moroccan Stew with Couscous,
194–95
in Mushroom Zucchini Quiche with
Rice Crust, 198–99
in Mushroom-Avocado Tofu
Scramble, 56
in Ratatouille, 266
in Sesame Tofu (Broiled Skewered)
with Hot Mustard Sauce, 174
in Squash, Sautéed Mixed, with
Cumin and Chili Powder, 268
in Tempeh Stir-Fried with Zucchini
and Red Bell Pepper, 213
in Tempeh with Eggplant and
Tomato, 215
in Tofu "Meatballs," 219
in Vegetable Salad, Roasted, 141–42
in Vegetable Stir-Fry, 272
in Vegetable Stock, 100

About the Authors

Diana Schwarzbein, M.D., graduated from the University of Southern California (USC) Medical School and completed her residency in internal medicine and a fellowship in endocrinology at Los Angeles County USC Medical Center. She founded The Endocrinology Institute of Santa Barbara in 1993. She sub-specializes in metabolism, diabetes, osteoporosis, menopause and thyroid conditions, subjects she lectures on frequently. She lives with her husband in Santa Barbara, California.

Nancy Deville is a writer of fiction and nonfiction with a talent for making science easy to read and understand. She recently completed a novel and screenplay about trafficking in women. She is currently at work on a second novel and a nonfiction book. She is a contributing writer on *Legacy: Secrets of Family Business Dynasties,* to be published by St. Martins Press. She lives with her husband in Santa Barbara, California.

Evelyn Jacob combines her love of cooking with her artistic talents. She is the former co-owner of the New York Bagel Factory of Santa Barbara and the founder and former director of Project Food Chain, a program that provides meals for people with AIDS and other life-challenging illnesses. She currently works as a private executive chef and caterer, as well as developing recipes for gourmet food companies. She lives with her husband and two sons in Carpinteria, California.

Diana Schwarzbein, M.D., Nancy Deville and Evelyn Jacob are also the authors of *The Schwarzbein Principle Cookbook.*

More Great Books from Dr. Schwarzbein

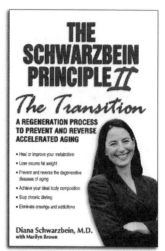
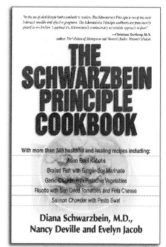